The Bible's Seven Secrets
to Healthy Eating

THE
Bible's
SEVEN SECRETS TO
Healthy
Eating

Joyce Rogers

CROSSWAY BOOKS • WHEATON, ILLINOIS
A DIVISION OF GOOD NEWS PUBLISHERS

The Bible's Seven Secrets to Healthy Eating

Copyright © 2001 by Joyce Rogers

Published by Crossway Books
              a division of Good News Publishers
              1300 Crescent Street
              Wheaton, Illinois 60187

Cover design: Liita Forsyth

Cover Photos: Foodpix®, EyeWire®, PhotoDisc®

Interior Illustrations: Liita Forsyth

First printing 2001

Printed in the United States of America

Unless otherwise designated, Scripture references are taken from the *New King James Version.* Copyright © 1982, Thomas Nelson, Inc. Used by permission.

Verses designated KJV are taken from the King James Version of the Bible.

Library of Congress Cataloging-in-Publication Data
Rogers, Joyce.
    The bible's seven secrets to healthy eating / Joyce Rogers.
       p.   cm.
    Includes bibliographical references and index.
    ISBN 1-58134-267-5
    1. Nutrition—Religious aspects—Christianity. 2. Food in the Bible.
3. Eating disorders—Religious aspects—Christianity. 4. Weight loss—
Religious aspects—Christianity. I. Title.
RA784.R625   2001
613.2—dc21   00-011619
                                                CIP

15	14	13	12	11	10	09	08	07	06	05	04	03	02	01
15	14	13	12	11	10	9	8	7	6	5	4			

Dedication

To my husband, Adrian, who has encouraged me along this twenty-year journey and who has frequently expressed appreciation for my efforts, for which I am extremely grateful.

To my children—Steve, Gayle, David, and Janice—who "endured" my extreme nutritional change of lifestyle in the beginning. I hope this book will influence them toward healthy lifestyles for their futures.

To my grandchildren—Renae, Angie, Rachel, Michael, Adrian, Jonathan, Andrew, and Stephen—who I trust one day will remember me not only for encouraging them to eat healthier diets, but for pointing them to Jesus, the Source of true spiritual satisfaction.

To my precious friend Juanita Dormer who recently went home to heaven after an extended bout with cancer. Through good nutritional practices, her life was greatly extended.

CONTENTS

ACKNOWLEDGMENTS

I am thankful to my husband, Adrian, who encouraged me to write this book. He read the manuscript and made valuable suggestions. He challenged me to think logically, helped me to examine biblical dietary principles, and has eaten without complaint and with real enjoyment whatever I set before him.

I owe a debt of gratitude to three doctors who reviewed my manuscript and provided valuable suggestions: Mark Castellaw, M.D., internist and Christian friend, who shared insights with me in my pursuit of prevention as a chief means of healthy living; Charles (Chuck) Hannaford, Ph.D., Christian clinical psychologist and friend, who kindly helped me in this exciting adventure; and Phillip L. Dowdle, D.D.S., dentist, who along with his wife, Evelyn, have been supportive friends of mine for more than twenty-five years and have practiced a lifestyle of healthy eating.

Thanks to Julia Flanagan, gifted editor and precious friend, who not only made invaluable suggestions and corrections to this book, but who was also genuinely interested in the subject of nutrition and was always excited about this project. Thanks, as well, for her creative design of the inside pages. And I thank Lila Bishop, editor at Crossway, for her valuable help.

I also owe a big thank you to my longtime friend Terri Nanney, who first introduced me to a more healthful way of eating. And I'm grateful to Terri and to her husband, Dr. Mike Nanney, M.D., for reviewing my manuscript.

And last but not least, I thank God for the bountiful riches in His Word that have been the guiding light in my journey of healthful eating. This lifelong adventure of getting to know and love Jesus has been entirely satisfying. "It is enough to see Jesus and go on seeing Him."[1]

PREFACE

It has been over twenty years since I was introduced to a healthier lifestyle of eating natural whole foods and following biblical dietary guidelines. I did not have a life-threatening disease, but I was extremely fatigued and susceptible to frequent colds and tension.

Today I have more energy than when I was much younger. I have far fewer colds and am in excellent all-round good health.

When I began this pilgrimage, I determined to adopt a more nutritional lifestyle as a means of prevention instead of a cure. I wanted to lead a productive life into my senior years. Since that time, nutrition has become a hobby to me. I'm constantly reading in this area and trying to improve the way I eat.

When I was first introduced to the "whole foods" way of life, I wanted to tell everyone. I thought they would be as receptive as I was. But I soon discovered that they weren't. It was then that I decided to be more low key and just talk with those who asked.

In recent years I have become more vocal again. I have felt a compulsion to at least share what I've learned, because a number of my close friends and acquaintances have either died or become ill with cancer and other serious diseases.

This book is a very brief introduction to the world of natural, whole foods and offers biblical insights into this subject. May it encourage you to seek truth for yourself. The first part of Hosea 4:6 says, "My people are destroyed for lack of knowledge." I have discovered that most Christians know far less about good nutrition than some members of false religions. Many food stores are replete with materials from New Agers and some false cults that emphasize a healthy lifestyle.

While this book is intended to be helpful, it does not make any claims for dramatic healing. It is meant to encourage a healthier lifestyle through a balanced diet of wholesome foods. Although healing sometimes occurs through God-given natural means, these suggestions are primarily given as a preventive measure for disease and as a prescriptive methodology for healthful living. One should always check with his or her doctor before making any drastic dietary changes.

The best time to begin a lifetime of healthful eating is when your children are babies. Train them early to like good things. Avoid using sweets and other not-so-good foods (i.e., candy, chips, cookies, and french fries) as baby-sitters or bribes.

Yes, it will take some added effort on your part. But it will be well worth it. I recently read a report about how the arteries of the young people in our nation are becoming clogged and how our children are becoming obese through unhealthy eating practices and lack of exercise (too much TV and Internet).

Dr. Kenneth Cooper, president of Cooper Clinic, has written a book entitled *Fit Kids!* He makes some statements that should make every parent stand up and take notice:

- More than one in five children ages six to seventeen are overweight. The number of "super-obese" children (20 to 30 percent overweight) has almost doubled in the past twenty years.

- Sixty percent of children have at least one modifiable risk factor for heart disease by age twelve.[1]

Even without these alarming statistics, it's just common sense that children should be eating healthful food and exercising regularly—like all of us! The U.S. Food and Drug Administration has some helpful literature and an interactive, informative web site that you should check out to get your child involved: http://vm.cfsan.fda.gov/~dms/educate.html.

At whatever age your children are, begin today. Of course, you must change your own eating habits, because you certainly can't expect your children to change without you! Why not try adopting a once-a-week dessert habit instead of dessert at every meal? Encourage your children with an award system for good eating habits. Whatever you can do to encourage healthy eating habits will pay high dividends—a longer and healthier life. Remember, begin today.

FAMILY MEALTIME "AROUND THE TABLE"

When you eat the labor of your hands, you shall be happy, and it shall be well with you. Your wife shall be like a fruitful vine in the very

*heart of your house, your children like olive plants all around your
table. (Psalm 128:2-3)*

My Childhood Home

The Bible speaks of family mealtime. In fact, children are pictured as
olive plants "around the table." I am a strong believer in and advocate
for family mealtimes. That is what I remember from my childhood.
We gathered around the big oak table for breakfast, suppertime, and
whenever everyone was present. Sunday dinner was always special when
we found ourselves "around the table."

My daddy was a man of few words; instead he taught much by his
example. At family mealtimes he taught many valuable lessons. We were
all seated before the meal began, which taught us family unity. He
taught punctuality by requiring that we all be on time. Our unity was
linked to reverence for God. To express that, we joined hands and
bowed our heads and hearts together to pray.

Another lesson I learned by quiet example was good manners.
Daddy never filled his plate first, but always passed the serving dishes
to Mama and then to us. We had good times around the table, too—
sharing jokes and experiences of the day.

Traditions Transferred

Family mealtime was a tradition Adrian and I brought into our home
when we got married. When our four children were still at home, you
would find us around the table whenever it was possible.

We continued most of those family mealtime traditions of my
childhood. When I hear of families who rarely eat together, it's hard
for me to believe it. I know it's difficult at times, but the busier we are,
the more important it is to gather around the table.

Family meals are worth the extra effort. Indeed, I didn't realize all
the lessons I was learning until I looked back at family mealtime. I
hope my children look back one day to lessons taught by quiet example sitting around the table.

Praying in the Empty Nest

There are just two of us now. We have a so-called empty nest. But we still hold hands and pray and thank our heavenly Father for His goodness, His mercy, and His grace.

I don't like it much when my husband has breakfast meetings, although I must "endure" a few. I give up our breakfast time reluctantly because it is our time for family prayer and worship. That's when Adrian and I pray for our children and grandchildren and those with special needs. Then we pray "around the world" as we hold hands "around the table."

So, if you come to breakfast at our house, you'll find us around the table fellowshipping and praying for those we know and love and for those we've never met but want to meet one day in God's house around His table.

More Nutritious Meals "Around the Table"

Mealtime has become more nutritious as the years have come and gone. Mama served the most nutritious meals she knew how to fix. And I "tried" my best with the knowledge that I had to feed my family with tasty things to build healthy bodies.

Now I have discovered a new level of nutrition, so you won't find some of the things that used to be passed around our table—sausage and gravy, bacon and white biscuits, doughnuts and Danish pastries. Instead you'll find whole wheat pancakes or waffles, oatmeal with fruit and honey, whole grain cereals with fresh fruit and nut topping, and sometimes an omelet filled with good things served with homemade whole wheat bread and honey. Now don't feel sorry for us, because we love what we eat and feel better than we ever have!

The purpose of our search for truth in the area of nutrition should primarily be to "glorify God in our bodies," not merely to look and feel good. These benefits will be by-products as we seek to please God and keep our bodies clean and fit as temples of the Holy Spirit.

> *Or do you not know that your body is the temple of the Holy Spirit who is in you, whom you have from God, and you are not your own? For you were bought at a price; therefore glorify God in your body and in your spirit, which are God's. (1 Corinthians 6:19-20)*

Above all, I want to point you to Jesus, the secret to true satisfaction. He is that Spring in the desert and the bread of life. His wisdom is sweeter than honey.

His Word is like spiritual milk and meat that enable us to grow stronger in our faith. His precious blood, shed on Calvary's cross, is even symbolized by the "blood" of the grape.

Good nutrition will give you a more vibrant physical life. Jesus will give you abundant eternal life. Look to Him to be your all in all.

INTRODUCTION

GOOD PROVISIONS IN A GOOD LAND

God promised seven good provisions to Abraham and his descendants in the good land of Canaan. And I believe that all of these provisions have literal and spiritual applications for us today.

This good land was bountifully created with brooks of water, grains, fruits, vegetables, oil, flocks, and herds. It was also flowing with milk and honey (see Deuteronomy 6:3; 8:7-10). As part of the promise, God challenged His people to keep His commandments, and they would enjoy His blessings as a result. If they forgot the Lord their God, they would perish. First Corinthians 10:6 says, "Now these things became our examples, to the intent that we should not lust after evil things as they also lusted."

Although much has been discovered in modern nutritional research, from which we can greatly benefit, God's Word provides timeless principles that can help clear up contradictions and confusion in this field of study.

It is the nature of God to want to meet the deepest needs of those He loves. This includes all of life's needs—those of the body, soul, and spirit. He is Lord of all, and the Scripture teaches that whether we eat or drink or whatever we do, we're to do all to the glory of God (see 1 Corinthians 10:31). I send this volume out with a prayer that your body, soul, and spirit will be nourished.

Just banish the thought that healthful foods don't taste good. Discover anew the taste of fresh fruits and vegetables; freshly baked whole grain bread with butter and honey; steaming lamb or beef stew with onions, potatoes, and carrots; broiled fish with roasted ears of corn; or chicken and brown rice with fresh stir-fried vegetables. Who would not want to enjoy good things to eat and abundant health at the same time?

Come now and let us examine these seven good things to eat and drink—God's wonderful provisions for our enjoyment and our health.

We'll look at practical applications for our health. Then we will gain spiritual insights from each of these seven provisions.

Did you know that seven is the perfect number? Perhaps it is not just a coincidence that there were seven divine provisions in this good land of bountiful blessings. Let's examine each one and see what applications they have to our lives.

1

Water

... a land of brooks of water,
of fountains and springs,
that flow out of valleys and hills.

DEUTERONOMY 8:7b

A LAND OF BROOKS OF WATER

I have traveled this good land that God's Word talks about. I've seen the waterfalls and pools, the brooks and streams that flow into the Jordan River and then flow into the beautiful blue Sea of Galilee.

How exciting to discover this precious, pure water when one has traveled through the desert or over the rocky hills. Nothing is so refreshing or satisfying as a cool drink of fresh water. Wouldn't you agree?

How precious and life-giving is water! It is so priceless that it is used as one of the chief symbols of Christ Himself. The Bible tells us that the Israelites in the wilderness "all drank the same spiritual drink. For they drank of that spiritual Rock that followed them, and that Rock was Christ" (1 Corinthians 10:4).

Jesus refers to Himself as living water in John 7:37-39:

On the last day, that great day of the feast, Jesus stood and cried out, saying, "If anyone thirsts, let him come to Me and drink. He who believes in Me, as the Scripture has said, out of his heart will flow rivers of living water." But this He spoke concerning the Spirit, whom those believing in Him would receive; for the Holy Spirit was not yet given, because Jesus was not yet glorified.

IMPORTANT FUNCTIONS OF WATER

It's amazing that we have so overlooked the value and importance of drinking water. Water is a necessity for life. Drinking sufficient water is one of the easiest and most important ways we can improve our health.

Water has many critical benefits, including helping keep us free from infections. Water also makes spinal fluid to cushion and control the nervous system. "It is necessary for all digestive, absorption, circulatory, and excretory functions, as well as for the utilization of the water-soluble vitamins."[1]

We think we have to add something to water—tea, coffee, carbonation, flavor, or sugar. But what we really need is to make a deliberate choice to return to plain old-fashioned water. And when our taste buds have made the adjustment, how much better everything will taste. Now I enjoy the true flavor of the food I eat. And I love the taste of good, pure water.

In addition:

- An average adult body contains about forty-five quarts of water.
- The temperature of the body is controlled through water.
- Water makes up 65 percent of the human body.
- Water makes up 92 percent of the blood of the human body.
- Water makes intestinal, gastric, saliva, and pancreatic juices.[2]
- Water prevents dehydration resulting in parched, dry skin, chronic constipation, and burning, irritating urine.
- Water holds all nutritive factors in solution and acts as a transportation medium to various parts of the body.
- Water keeps mucous membranes soft and free from friction.[3]

If we drink too little water, we will likely suffer from constipation and increase our risk of heat exhaustion or even heat stroke! Lack of water can also make us more susceptible to asthma attacks, dental disease, kidney stones, and urinary tract infections.

Consumer Reports on Health warns that if we don't monitor an adequate daily intake of water, we may be increasing our chances of getting a cold or even cancer. If we become dehydrated, we can also suffer from headaches, fatigue, lightheadedness, muscle cramps, and slightly dulled thinking.[4]

Paul Bragg, a world-famous physical fitness authority, said:

> I think that the excessively nervous person and/or the mentally upset person is so obsessed with his own worries and hang-ups that he just forgets to drink water and liquids of the right kind. Instead he dopes himself on alcohol, tea, coffee, and cola drinks. This complicates his nervous condition and burning, toxic acid forms in the stomach with no water to dilute it.
>
> So on top of his nervousness and depression, he suffers from sour acid stomach, heartburn, gas-bloat, and other miseries. Instead of drinking water, many people take aspirin, use cigarettes and other stimulants. Remember that the nerves need the correct amount of water to function properly and smoothly. We need to drink six to eight glasses of water each day. You can plainly see that it is possible to suffer from water starvation.[5]

WHAT KIND OF WATER SHOULD WE DRINK?

As in many areas, experts disagree over what kind of water we should drink. Some say we should drink mineral water from fresh, unpolluted springs. Others say we should drink distilled water without the minerals because the minerals in regular water cannot be absorbed in the body, they believe. Many people have installed water purifiers or distillers to help eliminate chlorine and other harmful additives.

Dr. Norman Walker recommends drinking distilled water because it helps to cleanse inorganic mineral deposits that are of no constructive value from the body. He writes that "distilled water collects the minerals discarded . . . originally collected from its contact with the earth and rocks."[6] The distilled water does not leach the organic minerals that your body uses.

Many people are totally oblivious to any benefits or harmfulness of different types of water and drink only according to taste. Our refrigerator has a purifier on its water dispenser; however, I drink distilled water whenever available. I would encourage you to read all sides of the story and then make your choice wisely. At any rate, you should drink lots of water!

Concerns About Water Quality

Most people assume that tap water is clean and healthy. They say, "If it's clear, it must be clean!" However, this may not be the case. Today we need to be concerned about the chlorine, pesticides, and parasites that may be in our tap drinking water.

Chlorine has long been added to public drinking water to kill disease-causing bacteria. But the levels of chlorine can be quite high, and some by-products of chlorine are known carcinogens.[7]

Something even more dangerous are the pesticides that may be present in our tap water. Pesticides are suspected of causing or contributing to breast and liver cancer. This is because the breast is made of fatty tissue, and toxins tend to accumulate in fatty tissue and the liver.

What About Carbonated Water?

Plain water is better than carbonated beverages for quenching your thirst and avoiding dehydration simply because you can drink more. According to Dr. Dean Edell: "Because the bubbles in carbonation take up room, an eight-ounce glass of plain water holds more water than an eight-ounce glass of carbonated water."

Dr. Edell does not think that carbonation leaches calcium from the bones—contrary to some opinions. However, he states that cola drinks may have a harmful effect on bones because of the phosphoric acid that is injected into the colas.[8] A chief problem with carbonation is that it causes abdominal bloating and gas.

Water from Other Sources

Many claim that they don't need to drink six to eight glasses of water each day because they eat lots of fruits and vegetables. I've heard people say that the coffee, juice, milk, etc., they drink gives them the liquid their body needs. This is not entirely true; these liquids cannot take the place of pure water. I do, however, want to add that juice can be a refreshing substitute for sodas.

Coffee, on the other hand, is another issue altogether. Like alcohol, caffeinated coffee is a diuretic and can cause a person to eliminate as much liquid as he or she consumes. It's best to avoid them both! Try drinking herbal teas instead. There are many varieties available.

SPIRITUAL APPLICATION

You Will Never Thirst Again

Jesus told the woman at the well that if she would drink of the water that He gave, she would never thirst again (see John 4:10). What a satisfying drink that was! She drank of this pure, sparkling Living Water, and she ran to get others to do the same! Truly, Jesus is a well of water springing up to everlasting life!

As the Deer Longs for Water

Thirst is used as a description of our longing after God. David had been hiding in the caves at En Gedi, an oasis in the desert. He had seen the deer leaping on the rocky hillside, searching for a drink from a clear, calm stream. He had seen the refreshment of that beautiful animal as it deeply drank to satisfy its thirst. And he saw in that scene a spiritual lesson.

David thirsted after God in a similar way. Psalm 42:1 says, "As the deer pants for the water brooks, so pants my soul for You, O God." David was physically thirsty. He longed for a drink from Bethlehem's well.

David was also spiritually thirsty. Psalm 63:1-2 says, "O God, You are my God; Early will I seek You; My soul thirsts for You; My flesh longs for You in a dry and thirsty land where there is no water. So I have looked for You in the sanctuary, to see Your power and Your glory."

Jesus, That Spring in the Desert

I had the privilege of visiting the oasis at En Gedi in the midst of the desert near the Dead Sea. I climbed the steep paths that passed by many fresh springs and flowing brooks. I finally arrived at the beautiful waterfall and pool at the very top. During the climb I was constantly reminded that Jesus is the Spring in the desert, the flowing River of Living Water, the heavenly drink from Bethlehem's well.

Jesus promises true satisfaction to each of us. Blessed fulfillment is ours when we thirst after righteousness (see Matthew 5:6). Won't you come to Him and drink? He is pure and fresh. He will satisfy your dry and thirsty soul!

> *But to the blessed cross of Christ one day I came*
> *Where springs of living water did abound.*
> —JOHN W. PETERSON

ASK YOURSELF

At the end of each chapter I'll ask you to evaluate yourself on a spiritual and practical level. First, the practical questions: "Am I drinking eight glasses of water every day? How does my complexion look? (Did you know that water flushes toxins out of your body and gives you a more radiant, clear complexion?) Am I substituting anything in the place of water— fruit juices, carbonated sodas, coffee, or tea?"

Now for some spiritual questions: "Do I long for Jesus as I do for a glass of water on a hot summer day? On those days when I feel that everything is going my way, is it because I am constantly filling myself with the goodness of Jesus, my Living Water? Could it be that I have satisfied my thirst with the things of this world so that I no longer desire a drink from the well of living water?"

A Bright Idea for Healthy Eating . . .

Invest in a large insulated water bottle. Each morning fill it up with cool water and keep it with you all day—in the car, at the office, everywhere you go. Sip on it all day to give your body what it's thirsting for!

Whole Grains

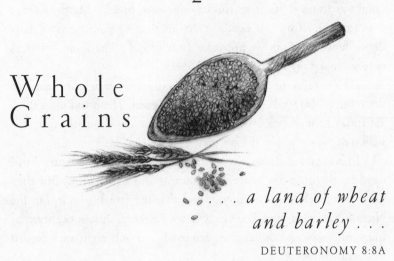

*. . . a land of wheat
and barley . . .*

DEUTERONOMY 8:8A

THE STAFF OF LIFE

Natural whole grains were abundant in the good land that God promised to the Israelites. Grains were literally the "staff of life" for these people. After the people cultivated their land and sowed their seed, God showered the crops with sunshine and rain. Then the harvest came.

We learn in the Bible that there were wheat harvests (Genesis 30:14) and barley harvests (Ruth 1:22). The barley harvests were in early spring around the time of Passover. The wheat harvests were about seven weeks later around Pentecost. Whole grain was a vital part of the diet of our spiritual ancestors.

The people in Bible times did not understand the benefits of having vitamins, minerals, protein, and fiber in their daily diets. However, they did not use refining processes that robbed the whole grains of most of their vitamins, minerals, and fiber. They used the whole grain.

The Great Grain Robbery

Prior to the 1900s most grain was milled locally, and bread was baked at home. At that time there was access to fresh whole grain flour. Only enough grain was ground to meet *daily* needs. Remember how Jesus taught us to pray? "Give us this day our *daily* bread" (Matthew 6:11, italics mine). While our Lord is teaching that we should have a daily dependence on Him, we note that Israeli food preparation practices ensured that daily bread was fresh bread.

Today's refining process produces a finer, more delicate-textured flour, but it also steals away the life of the grain. The bread most of us eat today provides calories but little food value—contributing to a nation of flabby, unhealthy people.

To make the situation worse, the food refiners claim to "enrich" this dead food with a few synthetic vitamins and a little iron. But they never give back the natural goodness that they steal from it. Dr. Joe Nichols has called this "The Great Grain Robbery." About twenty vitamins, minerals, and proteins are removed, and only eight are returned in a synthetic form.[1]

Wheat Germ and Bran

Two life-giving elements of the whole wheat kernel are removed in the refining process. They are the wheat germ and the bran. But what exactly are these elements, and why are they important to our diet?

Bran is the outer layer of the grain that contains the fiber. It is rich also in folic acid that helps prevent heart disease and in minerals—especially iron—and protein. The wheat germ is the richest source of the natural vitamins niacin, riboflavin, potassium, magnesium, iron, zinc, copper, manganese, and vitamins E and K. In addition, wheat germ is necessary for the absorption of vitamin A and for general vitality. And it is one of the best sources of the natural vitamin B complex and high-quality proteins. Now that's a mouthful of goodness!

THREE GREAT INGREDIENTS IN THE STAFF OF LIFE

Fiber

There's a lot of talk these days about the necessity of having fiber in our diets. Think of fiber as the skeleton of all plants, and the nourishment is inside the wall of fiber. Fiber is concentrated in the outer coats of grains such as wheat, barley, or corn.

In the same way that a sponge holds water when put into a glass, fiber holds water when in the colon. Because fiber acts in this way, it helps to protect against constipation that is basic to numerous diseases such as appendicitis, diverticulitis, hiatal hernia, hemorrhoids, varicose veins, heart disease, diabetes, obesity, large bowel cancer, and gallstones.

But all fiber is not the same. Did you know that the fiber in peas, beans, or apples is not the same kind of fiber you get in whole wheat bread? Many vegetables, as well as oat bran, barley, and nuts, contain soluble fiber that can be digested in the body. The fiber in whole wheat bread, however, is insoluble—the body cannot digest it. Both types of fiber are valuable.

Without going into too much detail, let me just say that soluble fiber attracts water and turns into gel during digestion. The rate of absorption of all the nutrients we need is slowed down by this fiber. On the other hand, insoluble fiber that we find in wheat bran, some vegetables, and whole grains works to speed the passage of foods in the digestive processes of our bodies. It also works to help us absorb the nutrients we need from the foods we eat. And it protects us from absorbing toxins, such as pesticides, that may come along with some foods.

Today's diets in the Western world are low in fiber. They are also very high in fat. The average American eats ten to fifteen grams of fiber per day, and yet the recommendation for older children, adolescents, and adults is twenty to thirty-five grams per day. Fiber is not just a good suggestion; it's a necessity for living a long, healthy life. It also helps to lower cholesterol.

We need to incorporate fiber-rich grains into our diet. And that means more brown rice, unrefined oats, barley, wheat, and corn. We need to get back to eating whole grain breads and whole grain pastas. Also, we need to cut down on our fat, sugar, and salt. When we do this, we'll reduce our risk of getting many diseases, such as breast and colon cancer, diabetes, high blood pressure, and heart failure.

Here's a good idea for your next trip to the grocery store. When you're looking at all the cereals and breads, read the labels! Check to make sure that these processed foods contain fiber-rich grains. And look elsewhere in the grocery for fiber-rich foods.

Legumes are a marvelous source of fiber. Whole wheat noodles provide two more grams of fiber per half-cup serving than regular noodles. Fruits and vegetables (which are covered in chapter 5) are also good sources of fiber. Many provide two to three grams of fiber per half-cup serving.

Whole potatoes (with the skins still on) are one of the most complete foods. But don't lather them with oodles of butter and sour cream. Try a little Dijon mustard with some low-fat yogurt. It's delicious and good for you!

Vitamin E

Whole grains are rich in vitamin E, a fat-soluble vitamin composed of compounds called tocopherols. Of these, alpha tocopherol is the most potent form of vitamin E and has the greatest nutritional and biological value. Tocopherols occur in the greatest concentrations in cold-pressed vegetable oils and all whole raw seeds, nuts, soybeans, and wheat germ.

Vitamin E is an antioxidant, which means it opposes oxidation—a natural process associated with aging and disease, including hardening of the arteries. It prevents saturated fatty acids and vitamin A from breaking down and combining with other substances that may become harmful to the body. It also helps reverse fibrocystic disease of the breast.

This vitamin has the ability to unite with oxygen and prevent it from being converted into toxic peroxide, leaving the red blood cells more fully supplied with vitamin E. Vitamin E plays an essential role in cellular respiration of all muscles, especially cardiac and skeletal muscles. It prevents blood clots from forming. It also aids in bringing nourishment to the cells, protecting the red blood cells from destruction.

Because aging in the cells is due primarily to oxidation, vitamin E is useful in retarding this process. It is also necessary for proper focusing of the eyes in the middle-aged person. It prevents scar formation. As a diuretic, it helps lower elevated blood pressure.

Vitamin E protects against the damaging effects of many environmental poisons in the air, water, and food. It protects the lungs and other tissue from damage by polluted air. It has a dramatic effect on the reproductive organs; it helps prevent miscarriages and increases male and female fertility. Research has also shown that vitamin E helps reduce the risk of Alzheimer's disease.

If you didn't know it before, you know it now: Vitamin E is one of the most essential components in a whole grain diet.

Vitamin B Complex

The vitamin B complex is another of the vital components of a whole grain diet that we need to consider. It is essential for health and energy, but the refining process of whole grains eliminates it. This is the "mystery" vitamin that is missing in refined white rice. The lack of it caused the disease beriberi. Today enough synthetic vitamin B is added to refined products to prevent this disease.

Vitamin B_6 is a water-soluble vitamin found in beans, nuts, legumes, eggs, meats, fish, whole grains, and fortified breads and cereals. It plays a role in the synthesis of antibodies in the immune system. It helps maintain normal brain function and acts in the formation of red blood cells. It is also required for the chemical reactions of proteins. Many symptoms are appearing in the population as a result of foods too low in this essential nutrient. Indeed, we are a fatigued, harried generation.

GRIND WHOLE GRAINS AND MAKE YOUR OWN BREAD

Every day I live, I continue to be impressed with the importance of including 100 percent whole wheat or multigrain bread in my diet. However, I didn't realize until I was well into my healthy lifestyle that even the whole wheat flour and bread that I bought in the health food store were missing many important vitamins.

"Clinical tests reveal that virtually all the vitamins stored inside a wheat kernel are oxidized within seventy-two hours."[2] What does that mean? It means that crucial nutrients our bodies need to fight aging and disease evaporate within three days of processing! All the more reason we need to incorporate fresh whole grains into our diet every day!

I can think of no better way to get God's whole grain goodness into our diets than to include fiber in our "daily bread." When you incorporate a daily dose of whole grain fiber into your diet, it's like giving yourself a free life insurance policy! Without it, your body is not getting what it needs to run most efficiently.

Several years ago I was visiting with my friend Linda, who served delicious homemade whole wheat bread each morning for breakfast. Her thirteen-year-old son baked the bread and even sold some each week for extra money. I was intrigued. She told me that she ground her own wheat berries. That was the secret to the lighter texture and delicious flavor. It also was the secret to preserving the nutrients in the flour.

I went home a "believer," and for some time I have been grinding my wheat berries and other grains and making my own whole grain bread. It's wonderful! Just ask my husband. I also make delicious, light whole wheat pancakes, which my husband loves. One of the secrets is the freshly ground flour. Another secret for great pancakes is to use buttermilk. They melt in your mouth. My favorite recipes for whole grain goodness are in the recipe section of this book.

If you're interested in grinding your own grains, take a few minutes and research the Internet for a supplier of grain mills (you can find some sites on my Internet Resource section at the end of the book). Also, you may want to purchase a mixer with a dough hook for making breads.

NO JUNK FOOD IN THIS GOOD LAND

God provided no junk food in this good land. We may think that these things are good; but the Bible never uses pies, candy, or cake to symbolize spiritual truths. To the contrary, in Proverbs 23:3 we read, "Do not desire [the ruler's] delicacies, for they are deceptive food." Christians are frequently deceived by these goodies.

I remember a situation where I had not been able to eat supper, and only dessert was being served. I was so hungry that I decided to try one of the delicious-looking dainties. When I took a bite, I realized it was truly a "deceitful dainty." It seemed the biggest piece of nothing I had ever eaten.

Although I occasionally indulge in birthday cake or some other tempting dessert, I enjoy hot, freshly baked homemade bread more than any "deceitful dainty" I used to crave. I believe anyone can change his or her eating habits to become healthier, but it takes retraining the taste buds! If I can do it, I know you can, too. Trust me—you'll be glad you did!

SPIRITUAL APPLICATION

The Bread of Life

Jesus is the Bread of Life. He said:

> *Most assuredly, I say to you, he who believes in Me has everlasting life. I am the bread of life. Your fathers ate the manna in the wilderness, and are dead. This is the bread which comes down from heaven, that one may eat of it and not die. I am the living bread which came down from heaven. If anyone eats of this bread, he will live forever; and the bread that I shall give is My flesh, which I shall give for the life of the world. (John 6:47-51)*

A few verses later Jesus told the Jews that they could have eternal life if they would eat His flesh and drink His blood. John 6:52-57 reads:

> *The Jews therefore quarreled among themselves, saying, "How can this Man give us His flesh to eat?" Then Jesus said to them, "Most assuredly, I say to you, unless you eat the flesh of the Son of Man and drink His blood, you have no life in you. Whoever eats My flesh and drinks My blood has eternal life, and I will raise him up at the last day. For My flesh is food indeed, and My blood is drink indeed. He who eats My flesh and drinks My blood abides in Me, and I in him. As the living Father sent Me, and I live because of the Father, so he who feeds on Me will live because of Me."*

This was offensive language to the Jews because they could not perceive the deep spiritual meaning behind Jesus' statement. But He was saying that they could sustain their spiritual lives only by feeding on Him.

Jesus, Our Staff of Life

Jesus is our Staff of Life. What do I mean by "staff"? In Bible times it meant "bread," which was baked from dough made of wheat flour that had been leavened and made into loaves. When we pray, "Give us this day our daily bread," we must remember that we are also asking Jesus to be our daily portion and our sustenance. We must come to Him and Him alone for everything we need to live the abundant life He has promised us.

It's sad but true that many of us have become accustomed to spiritual junk food. Instead of being satisfied completely with His whole, unrefined Word—looking to Him to be our life—we look to the shallow, self-centered experiences of others. Oh, that we would long for the Lord as the songwriter says:

Bread of heaven, Bread of heaven,
Feed me till I want no more.

ASK YOURSELF

Take a few minutes and ask yourself the following: "What does my food pantry look like? Is it stocked with sugary cereals and snack bars? Or is it stocked with whole wheat flour to make waffles, pancakes, or maybe a loaf of bread? How about oatmeal and bran to make a bowl of oatmeal or fresh bran muffins? How much fiber am I getting each day? Do I need to add more to maintain a healthy lifestyle?"

Now look deep into your heart and ask, "Am I feasting on the Bread of Life—getting my nourishment from His Word, finding strength in His promises and hope in His presence? Am I sharing His staff of life with others—my friends, neighbors, coworkers, and family? What about the grocery store clerk? My dry cleaner? My child's teacher?"

A Bright Idea for Healthy Eating . . .

Check food labels in the grocery store to make sure the foods you're buying are rich in fiber. Try to purchase foods that have four or more grams of fiber in each serving!

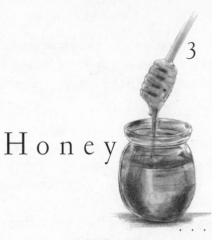

Honey

*. . . a land of olive oil
and honey.*

DEUTERONOMY 8:8

BEE-LIEVE IT OR NOT

Did you know that there is actually an admonition in the Bible to eat honey? The writer of Proverbs says, "My son, eat honey because it is good . . ." (Proverbs 24:13). Mentioned sixty-five times in the Bible (as "honey" or "honeycomb") and twenty times in the phrase "flowing with milk and honey," this delicious component of healthy eating is not only good, but it's good for you! In the days when the Bible was written, honey was the most common sweetener. Today it is of secondary importance because refined sugar is the world's most common sweetener.

Throughout the Bible you can read references to honey. Considered one of the "best gifts from God's land," honey was a customary present to someone of honor (see Genesis 43:11). Even in lean times when food was at a premium, honey was an essential staple in the biblical "pantry" (see 2 Samuel 17:29 and Isaiah 7:15, 22).

Though many of God's creations were burned as sacrifices, honey was not to be used as a burnt offering to God, but it was used instead as a "first fruits" offering to the Lord (see Leviticus 2:11; 2 Chronicles 31:5). The Word of God is compared to honey—noting that it is sweeter than even the sweetest thing the psalmist could imagine (see Psalm 19:10). You can also read about honey in the stories of Moses (Deuteronomy 32:13), Samson (Judges 14:8-14), Jonathan (1 Samuel 14:24-29), and John the Baptist (Matthew 3:4).

MANY DIFFERENT FLAVORS

First, let us consider the taste of honey. Maybe you have tried strong-tasting honey and said, "That's not for me." Perhaps you didn't realize that all honey is not the same.

Like cheese, honey has many flavors, ranging from dark and very strong to light and mild-tasting. There are blackberry, orange blossom, wildflower, and alfalfa honeys. Or choose from tupelo, apple, sage, or sweet clover. And this is just the beginning of the varieties of honey! There are more than 300 floral sources of honey in the United States alone![1] So if you're picky when it comes to honey, just take your pick.

GOOD AND GOOD FOR YOU

Honey not only tastes good; it is good for you. All honey is not created equal, however. When honey is heated in pasteurization, valuable enzymes, vitamins, and minerals are destroyed. Raw local honey is the best. In fact, some claim that this type of honey helps overcome allergies. If the honeycomb is included, you can know for certain that all the nutritional value is present.

"The mineral content of honey varies according to the source. The highest mineral content appears in dark honey, like buckwheat and heather, which have about four times as much iron as light honey, like clover, orange, and sage."[2] All honeys are alkaline in content, but scientists have discovered that the darker honeys have a higher alkaline level than the lighter ones.

It is difficult to determine the vitamin content of honey, which depends on whether it was produced in a hot, dry season or a cold, wet one. "It has been shown that the pollen of many flowers has a high vitamin C content; thus it has been assumed that the higher the pollen content, the more vitamin C it contains."[3]

Honey has been shown to contain vitamin B_2, which helps in the metabolism of carbohydrates. It also contains vitamin B6, important in protein metabolism and the prevention of skin diseases. And it contains B12, also important for metabolism and the formation of red blood cells and for the maintenance of the central nervous system. Other vitamins in honey are thiamin, riboflavin, niacin, biotin, pantothenic acid, folic acid, vitamin K, and carotene. "Vitamin K not only helps in blood clotting but also halts the formation of arid bacteria in the mouth, thus inhibiting tooth decay."[4]

Natural enzymes, including invertase, amylase, glucose oxidase, catalase, and acid phosphatase are valuable components of honey. Honey also contains proteins, calcium, sodium, potassium, magnesium, iron, chlorine, phosphorus, sulfur, and iodine salts, as well as many other mineral salts.

BALANCE, THE KEY TO VALUE

As in all areas of life, we find that the balance God creates is the best. If we will eat wholesome, natural foods in a well-balanced fashion, we will enjoy good health. However, if we eat too much of even a good thing such as honey, we will not be helping ourselves.

The same Bible that proclaims the value of honey also warns of using it too much. Proverbs 25:16 says, "Have you found honey? Eat only as much as you need, lest you be filled with it and vomit." And Proverbs 25:27a says, "It is not good to eat much honey." It's quite clear from God's Word that we are to be balanced consumers of honey. But did you know that the balance of the elements in honey is thought to be just as important for health as balance in eating honey? Any attempt to separate or extract one or more of these elements destroys this balance.

SPECIAL NOTE TO PARENTS

If you're a mom, perhaps you have thought about the great benefits of honey, but you read on the back of the container that honey wasn't good for your baby. The National Honey Board has this warning for parents:

> Your baby's tummy isn't ready for honey! Do not add honey to your baby's food, water, or formula. Do not dip your baby's paci-

fier in honey. Do not give your baby honey as medicine. Honey may contain bacterial spores that can cause infant botulism—a rare but serious disease that affects the nervous system of young babies (under one year of age). Botulism spores are common and may be found in dust, soil, and uncooked foods. Adults and children over one year of age are routinely exposed to, but not normally affected by, botulism spores. . . . The National Honey Board, along with other health organizations, recommends that honey not be fed to infants under one year of age.[5]

SUGAR—NOT SO GOOD

While the Bible declares that honey is good, modern man has found a cheaper and more refined substitute—white sugar. Sugar addicts around the world declare how g-o-o-d it is to the taste buds, but nutritional studies have shown that it is not so good for you.

This is bad news to those who think they cannot live without this sweet white stuff. They've even been fooled into thinking that sugar is listed among the essential nutrients. However, refined white sugar (or sucrose) and a number of other refined sugars have few or no nutrients. They have only calories, which are quick energy producers.

You may say, "Energy is essential; so sugar must be essential." The key lies in a definition of words and a clarification of terms. So many play the word game, and it's a very tricky game.

Don't believe everything you read, especially in the advertisements for not-so-good products. The proponents of sugar will lead you to believe that sucrose (or white sugar) is in the same category of carbohydrates as whole grains, whole potatoes, and fresh fruits. Yes, sugar is a carbohydrate, all right. However, it has been stripped of all its vital minerals and vitamins, especially the vitamin B complex, which is essential to the digestion of sucrose. When the vitamin B complex isn't present, the body is robbed of these precious vitamins in order to digest the sugar.

On April 12, 1973, three prominent doctors, two of them representing the American Medical Association's Council on Food and Nutrition, were testifying before a Senate Committee on nutrition and human need as to whether sugar was a nutrient or an anti-nutrient. It was a battle of finely defined words.

Some months later, a five-member arbitration panel of the National Advertising Review Board found that the claim that sugar was a nutrient was without foundation. The sugar pushers promised to stop making the claim until they could back it up. However, millions more people were misled before the sugar producers' ad was suspended.[6]

Sucrose or white sugar is responsible for many modern-day ills. First, and without question, it is related to obesity. And to make matters worse, the obese are more disposed to diabetes, which is linked to arteriosclerosis, blindness, Parkinson's disease, and other diseases.

Diabetes is due to altered metabolism, which causes the high blood sugar characteristic of this disease. Diabetes is the third highest cause of death in the United States. For those with a hereditary predisposition to diabetes, the effect of sugar could be much worse. Tragically, this disease has a very low recovery rate. In recent years the incidence of Type II diabetes has increased due to obesity and diet.

In 1923 a Canadian physician, Frederick Banting, received the Nobel prize for discovering a way to extract the insulin hormone (of which the average human pancreas excretes an adequate supply). He proved that this hormone could control the abnormal amounts of blood sugar that made diabetes mellitus a slow killer.[7]

But diabetes doesn't have to kill if caught in the early stages. Diabetics, under the close supervision of a doctor, can add many years to their lives if they adhere to a strict diet, which includes the restriction of sucrose or white sugar. If only we could prevent this terrible killer before it strikes, instead of trying to control it afterward.

Its sister disease, hypoglycemia (or low blood sugar), is also associated with this not-so-good product called sugar. Many with this condition suffer from fatigue, nervousness, and dizziness, and are thought to be hypochondriacs when, in fact, many of these people have low levels of glucose in their blood. Dr. Seale Harris in 1924 discovered that hypoglycemia is caused by excessive insulin.[8]

It's best to leave white sugar alone or have it only occasionally. Remember what this chapter is all about? Substitute honey for sugar—but then don't eat too much honey either!

Natural sugars are found in delicious fruits such as apples, oranges, peaches, bananas, plums, grapes, mangos, papayas, strawberries, blueberries, watermelons, cantaloupes, and many others. Not only are they sweet, but they are also powerhouses of vitamins, minerals, and enzymes. And eat the skins of most of them (wash them with soap and water first to remove pesticides). You'll benefit from the fiber!

SUBSTITUTING HONEY FOR SUGAR

Because honey packs a lot of sweetness in every single drop, you can use less honey than sugar to achieve the same sweetness in your favorite recipes. The National Honey Board offers the following guidelines:

> To substitute honey for sugar in recipes, start by substituting honey for up to half of the sugar called for. If the recipe calls for two cups of sugar, try one cup of sugar and three-fourths cup honey. When baking with honey, remember the following:

> - Reduce any liquid called for by one-fourth cup for each cup of honey used.
> - Add one-half teaspoon of baking soda for each cup of honey used.
> - Reduce oven temperature by 25°F to prevent over-browning.[9]

SPIRITUAL APPLICATION

Seeking Your Own Glory

Earlier in this chapter, I quoted the first half of Proverbs 25:27. Now let's look at the second half of that verse: "It is not good to eat much honey; *so to seek one's own glory is not glory*" (italics mine). Eating too much of this good sweetener is compared to searching out your own glory.

You may be a very "sweet" person. But if you dwell on it and attempt to let others know how sweet you are, you will be sickening to other people. Proverbs instructs us, "Let another man praise you, and not your own mouth; a stranger, and not your own lips" (Proverbs 27:2).

Like Wisdom to Your Soul

The Bible compares honey to wisdom. Proverbs 24:13-14 says, "My son, eat honey because it is good, and the honeycomb which is sweet to your taste. So shall the knowledge of wisdom be to your soul. If you have found it, there is a prospect, and your hope will not be cut off."

If you find wisdom, you will have a wonderful future full of hope. Just as a person is nourished and built up by honey, likewise will he or she be nourished and built up by wisdom. Yes, how sweet it is to possess wisdom.

The Judgments of the Lord

Elsewhere in the Bible we read that the Lord's judgments are sweeter than honey. "The fear of the LORD is clean, enduring forever; The judgments of the LORD are true and righteous altogether. More to be desired are they than gold, yea, than much fine gold; sweeter also than honey and the honeycomb" (Psalm 19:9-10).

If correct judgments are made, we must possess wisdom. If true justice prevails, it is pleasing and we are satisfied. However, if there is an injustice, an unfair decision, or a wrong verdict—immediately it causes bad feelings. If the problem is not corrected, it can lead to great bitterness of soul. Homes can be divided, friendships severed, and governments destroyed through a lack of justice.

Human judgment is perverted. We don't evaluate as God does. Oftentimes we add two plus two and get five. Unless God and His Word guide us, there will always be imperfect judgment. We must align our wills to His and submit to His judgments in all things. Indeed, the judgments of the Lord are true and altogether right. They are sweeter than honey and the drippings of the honeycomb.

God fed His children in the wilderness with honey from the rock (Deuteronomy 32:13), and He rained down manna from heaven that had the taste of honey (Exodus 16:31). We must come to our Lord, the Rock of our salvation. There is plenty of honey there—sweetness for our souls. We must come to our Lord—the Manna who came down from heaven. He will nourish us and satisfy us with His sweetness.

ASK YOURSELF

On a practical level, "Am I eating too much sugar? If I had recorded everything I ate for the last week, what would it show? Doughnuts? Sweet rolls? Cookies? Cakes? What dessert can I prepare this week, substituting honey for sugar? What can I do, even today, that would make a difference in the amount of sugar I've been eating?"

Now search your heart and ask, "What's my witness been like this week? Could someone compare me to the sweetness of honey? Or have I been more like the sour juice of a lemon? Am I delighting in God's Word the way I would delight in a sweet honey bun? Or am I viewing the precepts of the Lord as hardships?"

A Bright Idea for Healthy Eating . . .
Honey is not only a delicious alternative to sugar, but it is oh so good for you! Substitute it in your next recipe for a cake, cookies, or cobbler.

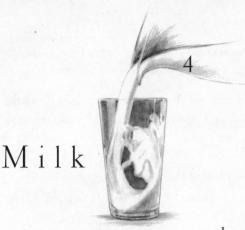

Milk 4

. . . a land flowing with milk and honey.

DEUTERONOMY 6:3

A LAND FLOWING WITH MILK AND HONEY

Throughout the Bible we note that milk was one of the staples as well in the diet of the Israelites. Milk was also a part of the meal Abraham served to the angels who visited him and Sarah to tell them that they were going to have a child in their old age (see Genesis 18:1-8).

The Bible mentions three types of milk—milk from cows, goats, and sheep (see Isaiah 7:21-22, Proverbs 27:27, and Deuteronomy 32:14). There are also references to eating butter (Proverbs 30:33) and cheese (Job 10:10; 2 Samuel 17:29). Curds of cow's milk are mentioned in Deuteronomy 32:14 (NASB) and Isaiah 7:15 (NASB). This was probably similar to our plain yogurt.

I visited a modern-day Bedouin tent in the Holy Land and observed yogurt being made in a big leather pouch hanging in the sun. As in Bible times, they still believe in the benefits of this dairy food.

The Bible also mentions milk in Deuteronomy 32:12-14:

So the LORD alone led him [Jacob], and there was no foreign god with him. He made him ride in the heights of the earth, that he might eat the produce of the fields. He made him draw honey from the rock, and oil from the flinty rock; curds from the cattle, and milk of the flock, with fat of lambs; and rams of the breed of Bashan, and goats, with the choicest wheat; and you drank wine, the blood of the grapes.

God brought Jacob while in the desert many good things from the good land, including milk and honey. Indeed God is our Jehovah Jireh—our Almighty Provider!

A CONTROVERSY ABOUT MILK

Many claim that milk is the most easily digested food. In fact, milk is necessary for a baby to grow up healthy and strong. But did you know that there is a controversy about milk and dairy products for adults? The dietary guidelines, fat content, calcium benefits, as well as the problem of lactose intolerance and respiratory disease issues are all up for debate these days.

Some say a gland that handles milk in the human body stops functioning when people reach a certain age, and adults should not drink it. Others say milk benefits are a matter of race and age. Motivated by the "Got milk?" ad campaign during the late 1990s, the Physicians Committee for Responsible Medicine issued this statement in a press release dated June 1, 1999:

> African-Americans and males in general have a much lower risk of osteoporosis, and there is no evidence that adding extra calcium—from milk or anything else—is helpful for these groups. Indeed, nearly all studies that have examined calcium intake have specifically excluded African-Americans due to differences in bone density. . . . Data in older women show that milk-drinkers have as many (or possibly even more) fractures as women who avoid milk.[1]

The Director of the American Council on Science and Health, Dr. Ruth Kava, countered with this rebuttal:

> Rather than helping, PCRM's extremist stance on milk and dairy products does a real disservice to members of minority groups. Women in these groups, and especially young women, should be told of the necessity of including sources of calcium in their diets—and should be told that dairy products are excellent sources of calcium. Furthermore, because hypertension occurs disproportionately in members of some minority groups, to warn such people away from valuable sources of calcium is to offer advice that is potentially detrimental to their health.[2]

Homogenization of Milk

And the debate continues on other grounds. Some say that homogenized milk is not good for you. Indeed, they may have a point. Dr. Rex Russell in his book *What the Bible Says About Healthy Living* points to Proverbs 30:33, which mentions the churning of milk. He says, "By biblical definition homogenized dairy products may no longer be milk, because churning homogenized milk won't bring forth butter."[3]

So is milk good for you? And if so, what kind? Some say that goat's milk is better for you than cow's milk. The molecular structure of goat's milk is closer to that of human milk. Goat's milk also contains casein, the allergy-triggering protein found in cow's milk. In addition, lactose (milk sugar) is present in similar amounts in both milks.

As for cow's milk, many tout skim or low-fat milk. However, vitamins A, D, E, and K are fat-soluble and cannot be adequately absorbed into the body without fat, so some fat is essential.

In my opinion, these questions about milk are not adequately answered. Until they are, I still consider milk products to be one of the chief sources for calcium, which is so essential for the building of healthy bones. Milk is also a rich source of protein, vitamin D, and vitamin B riboflavin that helps maintain your energy level.

One Answer to the Milk Controversy

Dr. Paavo Airola, in his book *How to Get Well*, states, "The answer to the milk controversy is simple: both sides are right! Milk is an excellent food for those who are milk-tolerant, and poison for those who are not."[4]

Dr. Robert D. McCracken, anthropologist at the University of Public Health, identifies those who are milk-tolerant and those who are not:

> Descendants of the countries and the ancestors [from Europe and the Middle East] who historically herded dairy animals and traditionally lived on a lactose-rich diet (milk, cheese, etc.) are usually tolerant to milk. Their intestines contain plenty of the enzyme lactose, which breaks down milk sugar into a form that the body can use.
>
> Conversely, those whose ancestors [from Africa, China, Philippines, New Guinea, India, Australia, or Alaska/Canada] never or seldom used milk as a major element of the diet are usually intolerant to milk because their intestines do not contain sufficient lactose.[5]

Dr. Airola, however, recommends using only uncontaminated raw milk from healthy animals. He believes that the pasteurized milk we buy in our stores is loaded with toxic drugs, chemicals, and residues of pesticides, herbicides, and detergents, making it unsuitable for human use. He, therefore, recommends using milk in its soured form—yogurt, kefir, acidophilus milk, or regular clabbered milk. He also believes that goats' milk is better than cows' milk.[6]

YOGURT AND OTHER CULTURED DAIRY PRODUCTS

Some claim that yogurt and cultured dairy products, including buttermilk, are really the healthy route to go. They say that these cultured dairy products contain the "friendly bacteria" that are absolutely essential for healthy intestines. When people take antibiotics, these "friendly bacteria" are destroyed, so it's a good idea to take yogurt or acidophilus supplements to restore the "friendly bacteria" to the intestines.

Yogurt contains the vitamin B complex and has a higher percentage of vitamins A and D than does the milk it's made from, and yogurt is also high in protein. This beneficial yogurt turns the "friendly bacteria" into a natural antibiotic. If the living cultures in yogurt have been destroyed, the product can no longer be considered true yogurt!

Note here the nutritional composition of low-fat plain yogurt. The "Percentage Daily Values" were recently set by the United States government.[7]

THE NUTRITIONAL COMPOSITION OF
LOW-FAT PLAIN YOGURT

	Per 100 g	1 cup (227 g)	% Daily
Calories	50.00	113.5	6
Protein (g)	4.30	9.8	20
Carbohydrate (g)	4.80	10.90	4
Fat (g)	1.10	2.5	4
Cholesterol (mg)	4.00	9.1	3
Calcium (mg)	173.00	393.0	39
Riboflavin (mg)	0.18	41.00	24
Phosphorus (mg)	111.00	252.0	25

How to Incorporate Yogurt into Your Healthy Eating

- For a fruit smoothie, combine 1/2 cup plain yogurt with 1/2 cup diced ripe fruit (i.e., banana, peach, or strawberries) and one or two ice cubes in a blender. Puree until smooth. You could use partially thawed frozen fruit instead of ice cubes.

- Combine 1/2 cup plain yogurt with one mashed ripe avocado, 1/4 cup diced tomato, and chili powder to taste. Serve as a dip with tortilla chips or topping for tacos, enchiladas, or hamburgers.

- Top broccoli, brussels sprouts, or asparagus with plain yogurt and sprinkle with minced fresh dill and chopped cashews.

- Top borscht, gazpacho, or cream of tomato soup with a dollop of plain yogurt and minced chives.[8]

- Top baked potato with plain yogurt mixed with a little Dijon mustard.

THE BONE DISEASE—OSTEOPOROSIS

The Facts

"Sometime between the ages of thirty and forty your bones will probably begin to lose the calcium that makes the bones strong."[9] And before you know it, you may suffer from the "silent disease"—osteoporosis. It is called this because you may not notice that you have any of the symptoms. It is a disease that thins and weakens bones to the point that they break easily—especially bones in the hip, spine, and wrist. About twenty-five million Americans have osteoporosis—80 percent are women.

The rate of bone loss is slow at first, whether you are male or female. But if you are female, the picture changes dramatically around the time of menopause. Suddenly your body experiences a sharp drop in estrogen, which helps to protect the bones by keeping calcium in them. Now the rate of bone loss jumps. The problem starts to become obvious in the form of broken bones.

Osteoporosis is responsible for more than 1.5 million fractures annually, including 300,000 hip fractures, approximately 700,000 vertebral fractures, 250,000 wrist fractures, and more than 300,000 fractures at other sites. The burden of health care costs due to osteoporotic fractures is estimated to be $13.8 billion per year.[10]

For years it was believed that the bones lost calcium if there was not enough calcium in our diets. The National Dairy Council is the primary spokesperson for this point of view, and the solution they propose is for us all to drink more milk and eat more dairy products.

The Factors Leading to Osteoporosis

Excess Dietary Protein. Though some may disagree, John Robbins says, "Osteoporosis is, in fact, a disease caused by a number of things, the most important of which is excess dietary protein. . . . The correspondence between excess protein intake and bone resorption is direct and consistent. Even with very high calcium intakes, the more excess protein in the diet, the greater the incidence of negative calcium balance, and the greater the loss of calcium from the bones."[11]

The more protein in our diet, the more calcium we lose, regardless of how much calcium we consume. One of the nation's leading medical authorities on dietary associations with disease, Dr. John McDougall, says, "I would like to emphasize that the calcium-losing effect of protein on the human body is not an area of controversy in scientific circles. The many studies performed during the past 55 years consistently show that the most important dietary change that we can make if we want to create a positive calcium balance that will keep our bones solid is to decrease the amount of proteins we eat each day."[12]

An Acid pH of the Blood. It is essential for the blood to maintain a neutral pH. If the blood becomes too acidic, we will die. If our diets contain a lot of acid-forming foods, then the body withdraws calcium from the bones and uses this alkaline mineral to balance the pH of the blood.

Meat is one of the most acid-forming of foods, and hence it causes calcium to be drawn from the bones to restore the pH balance. Now I'm not saying that you should eliminate meat from your diet, but I strongly encourage you to decrease your consumption of it. Most fruits and vegetables generally yield an alkaline ash, and so they require no depletion of calcium stores from the bones to maintain the neutrality of the blood.[13]

Too Much Phosphorus. The body's ability to absorb and utilize calcium depends on the amount of phosphorous in the diet. But today's generation is over-indulging in foods such as meat and soft drinks that are high in phosphorus.

In one study young women maintained a positive calcium balance when their diets provided 1500 milligrams of calcium and 800 milligrams of phosphorous per day. But when the phosphorous intake was raised to 1400 milligrams a day, the women went into negative calcium balance, even though their calcium intake had not been reduced.[14]

Other Contributing Factors to Osteoporosis

People are more susceptible if they

- are small, light-skinned Caucasian women.
- have borne no children or have had their ovaries removed.
- fail to get enough exercise.
- consume soft drinks (these are very high in phosphorous).
- consume junk food, excess salt, and acid-forming foods.
- are smokers.
- use certain anti-convulsant medications.[15]

AND

- have a family history of osteoporosis.
- have an early menopause.[16]

Preventative and Corrective Measures to Fight Osteoporosis

To discover whether you have osteoporosis, get a thorough medical examination, including a bone scan at your doctor's recommendation. There are new non-hormonal drug therapies available that will assist in building bone mass.

Of course, these measures cannot take the place of a healthy diet that should include a recommended balance of calcium, vitamin D, magnesium, and so on. A National Institute of Health panel recommends the following daily calcium levels (in milligrams) as protection against osteoporosis:

Women aged 25-50 need 1,000 milligrams a day, while women over 50 need 1,500. The only exceptions are women who take estrogen. NIH recommends 1,000 milligrams of calcium a day for this special group.[17]

Although I believe it is essential to get enough calcium in the diet, that is not the whole story. It is important to have good sources of phosphorus, magnesium, and vitamin D. Phosphorus assists in the metabolism of dairy products and acts as a reservoir for metabolic energy. Make sure the phosphorus you get equals half the amount of calcium you take in each day. Also, you'll need to know that magnesium interacts with calcium and with nutrients such as potassium, vitamin B6, and boron, which aid calcium absorption.

Dairy products, we know, contain calcium. In addition, you can get calcium from green leafy vegetables, broccoli, tofu, and other soy products.

According to *Smart Medicine for Healthier Living*, here are some other guidelines to help you fight this crippling disease:

- Limit your salt intake. Salt not only contributes to high blood pressure, but it also increases the likelihood of osteoporosis.

- Monitor your caffeine consumption carefully (or better yet, avoid caffeine entirely). It has been shown that women who drink more than two cups of regular coffee or caffeinated sodas per day suffer a loss of bone density that can lead to bone fractures later in life.

- Exercise! Regular weight-bearing exercise can stop, or at least slow, bone loss in postmenopausal women. Half an hour of jogging, aerobics, climbing stairs, or brisk walking daily is sufficient.

- Don't smoke. Smoking is a proven risk factor associated with a whole host of diseases, including osteoporosis.[18]

TEENAGE DIETARY HABITS HARD ON BONES

Although a lot of attention is being given to the amount of calcium being lost by the middle-aged and older woman, an even greater problem is the failure to absorb and utilize calcium during adolescence when bone development reaches its height. No bones about it, kids and teens can't do without it. Research sponsored by the National

Institute of Child Health and Human Development (NICHD) has shown that a "window of opportunity" exists to add to the bone bank during the teen years.

NICHD researchers have found that supplementing the daily diets of girls ages twelve to sixteen with an extra 350 milligrams of calcium produced a 14 percent increase in their bone density, in comparison to the girls who did not take supplements. If this increase in bone density could be maintained, its impact would be striking. For every 5 percent increase in bone density, the risk of later bone fracture declines by 40 percent. It is becoming increasingly evident that adequate calcium intake is critical during adolescent years.[19]

CALCIUM: WHO GETS ENOUGH?

Age Group	Percent Getting the 1989 RDA
Under 5 (males and females)	45.4
Males (6-11)	53.3
Males (12-19)	35.1
Males (20-29)	45.0
Females (6-11)	43.1
Females (12-19)	14.4
Females (20-29)	17.8

Source: USDA Continuing Survey of Food Intakes by Individuals, 1994. This survey was evaluated using 1989 Recommended Dietary Allowance (RDA). New calcium guidelines, Dietary Reference Intakes, were issued in August 1997 and generally set a higher intake standard.

The daily lifestyle of teenagers includes many of the contributing factors to osteoporosis. We should challenge them with the admonition in 1 Corinthians 6:19-20: "Or do you not know that your body is the temple of the Holy Spirit who is in you, whom you have from God, and you are not your own? For you were bought at a price; therefore glorify God in your body and in your spirit, which are God's."

As we remind teenagers to keep their bodies as temples of the Holy Spirit, we should likewise educate them as to the dangers that accompany these bad habits. Also we should instruct them in the basics of good nutrition and how this will benefit them for years to come.

A NOTE TO NURSING MOMS

Mothers' milk is the best milk for babies. It's no secret that this was God's design (see Exodus 2:1-10; 1 Samuel 1:21-23; Psalm 22:9; 1 Thessalonians 2:7; Isaiah 49:15-16; Luke 11:27-28). Adrian and I have four children and eight grandchildren. Most of them were fed ho-*mama*-nized milk for months. I know that nursing is difficult or impossible for some. But if at all possible, consider God's original plan. The following is from *God's Vision for Families,* a study manual about raising children:

> The best way to keep your baby healthy is to give it the perfect food that God has planned. Cow's milk is a perfect food—but only for cows! It was never intended for human babies! The cow is a big animal with four stomachs. It weighs about 90 lbs. at birth and in only two years it is a whopping 2,000 lbs. This is not the kind of food that is required for the human baby who weighs about 6-8 lbs. at birth and is only 100-200 lbs. twenty years later!
>
> The baby uses 100 percent protein from the mother's milk. Less than 50 percent can be absorbed from cow's milk or formula so that baby has to take twice as much, which is extra work on the kidneys. . . . Breast milk contains up to 10 times more essential vitamins than cow's milk. This difference is reduced when cow's milk is diluted and reduced further when the formula is heated. The immunity that breast milk affords lasts long after the child is weaned. Breastfed babies do not suffer from constipation, as breast milk forms a soft curd in the baby's stomach.[20]

MY PERSONAL CONCLUSION

I'm not going to stop enjoying milk and other dairy products unless further evidence comes in. However, as I mentioned in the last chapter about honey, it makes sense to avoid overdoing it on any good thing.

I use a lot of yogurt because what I've studied makes sense. In fact, sometimes I even make my own. I also take an acidophilus capsule every day. These are available in powder form and contain the "friendly bacteria" found in yogurt.

If you don't like the taste of plain yogurt, mix it with fruit and/or honey. Or try some on a baked potato instead of sour cream. Use it instead of mayonnaise in fruit salad or use half yogurt and half mayonnaise.

Here's an observation: Most commercial yogurts are not as healthy as they claim to be. Look on the label for the ingredients. If they list any "thickeners" (i.e., modified corn starch, gelatin, tapioca starch), that means they haven't gone through the hours of processing that makes true yogurt. Note also where sugar comes in that list. Often it is the next ingredient after milk, which makes this a high-sugar item.

SPIRITUAL APPLICATION

As Newborn Babes

The Bible instructs us: "As newborn babes, desire the pure milk of the word, that you may grow thereby" (1 Peter 2:2). New believers in the faith are like newborn babies. They are hungry and dependent. And the Word of God is their spiritual nourishment. The purpose for feeding on the milk of the Word is to grow spiritually.

The milk of the Word is the easily digested spiritual food of the Bible. It includes learning the basics of God's Word—salvation, baptism, prayer, Bible study, the Second Coming of Jesus, and the filling of the Holy Spirit.

Carnal Christians

Sometimes these baby Christians stay just that—baby Christians. We call them "carnal Christians" because they are spiritual babies whose growth has been stunted. They've never eaten the solid food of the Word. They haven't gone beyond the basics in the Christian life. And they aren't able to lead others to Christ, to teach others, or to trust God in difficult circumstances. These are the people Paul is talking about in 1 Corinthians 3:1-3:

> *And I, brethren, could not speak to you as to spiritual [people] but as to carnal, as to babes in Christ. I fed you with milk and not with solid food; for until now you were not able [to receive it,] and even now you are still not able; for you are still carnal. For where [there are] envy, strife, and divisions among you, are you not carnal and behaving like [mere] men?*

Hebrews 5:12-14 also mentions these believers:

For though by this time you ought to be teachers, you need someone to teach you again the first principles of the oracles of God; and you have come to need milk and not solid food. For everyone who partakes only of milk is unskilled in the word of righteousness, for he is a babe. But solid food belongs to those who are of full age, that is, those who by reason of use have their senses exercised to discern both good and evil.

Yes, it is clear that God's Word exhorts new believers to drink that spiritual milk so they can grow up.

ASK YOURSELF

On the practical side of things, "Am I getting the calcium I need each day to build strong bones and prevent osteoporosis? How am I getting my calcium—by eating high-fat cheese-laden pizza and sugary fruit-filled yogurts or by drinking low-fat milk and mixing low-fat plain yogurt with fruit? What changes can I make in my diet today to make sure I get my calcium without adding extra calories or fat?"

It's time now to ask, "Do I hunger after the pure milk and meat of God's Word? Am I hungering and thirsting after righteousness? Do I know that the sustenance of my body and soul are completely dependent upon my Father in heaven to provide for me? Am I the carnal Christian that the Bible speaks about? What am I feeding my mind and body every day—things that build me up or tear me down?"

A Bright Idea for Healthy Eating . . .

Soy milk is a healthy alternative to cow's milk. Because of its health benefits and long shelf life, it is a practical addition to your cupboard. Try it in your next recipe instead of cow's milk.

Fruits and Vegetables

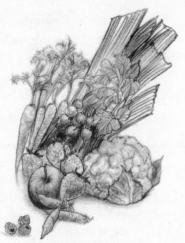

a land of . . .
vines and fig trees
and pomegranates . . .

DEUTERONOMY 8:8

. . . let them give us vegetables to eat
and water to drink.

DANIEL 1:12

THE GARDEN OF EDEN

On the third day of creation, God created fruits and vegetables as the
primary source of nutrition for His creatures, including mankind.

> *Then God said, "Let the earth bring forth grass, the herb that yields*
> *seed, and the fruit tree that yields fruit according to its kind, whose*
> *seed is in itself, on the earth"; and it was so. And the earth brought*
> *forth grass, the herb that yields seed according to its kind, and the*
> *tree that yields fruit, whose seed is in itself according to its kind. And*
> *God saw that it was good. (Genesis 1:11-12)*

Close your eyes and imagine what it would have been like in the Garden of Eden—to simply walk through that garden and pick greens for a salad, pull off ears of corn for dinner, and pluck a juicy orange for a snack. It must have been glorious—truly a paradise!

John Calvin made this comment about God's great goodness in creating fruits and vegetables for us to enjoy:

> When [God] says, "Let the earth bring forth the herb which may produce seed, the tree whose seed is in itself," He signifies not only that herbs and trees were then created, but that, at the same time, both were endued with the power of propagation, in order that their several species might be perpetuated.
>
> Since, therefore, we daily see the earth pouring forth to us such riches from its lap, since we see the herbs producing seed, and this seed received and cherished in the bosom of the earth till it springs forth, and since we see trees shooting from other trees; all this flows from the same Word.
>
> If therefore we inquire, how it happens that the earth is fruitful, that the germ is produced from the seed, that fruits come to maturity, and their various kinds are annually reproduced; no other cause will be found, but that God has once spoken, that is, has issued His eternal decree; and that the earth, and all things proceeding from it, yield obedience to the command of God, which they always hear.[1]

God, in His loving care for His children, created plants with life-giving nutrition for us in the Garden of Eden. From each plant we get more plants. The plants that He created contain seeds to provide us with a continued supply of His bountiful provision. It is a testimony to His power, His faithfulness, and His love that all things are created and sustained by His omnipotent hand.

In Proverbs 15:17 we are introduced to the Hebrew word for vegetables—*yârâq*. This verse is especially poignant for this book, "Better is a dinner of *yârâq* [vegetables] where love is, than a fatted calf with hatred." The Hebrew word *zêroâ,* is another word for vegetables in the Old Testament and is used in the references of Daniel chapter one, which we'll discuss later in this chapter.

Fruits are mentioned throughout the Bible; the Hebrew word for fruit is *peri,* and the Greek word for fruit is *karpos.* The fruits most often mentioned in Scripture are the grape, pomegranate, fig, olive, and apple. Each time we read about fruit in the New Testament, whether figuratively or literally, a form of the same word *karpos* is used. The only exceptions are in Matthew 26:29, Mark 14:25, and Luke 22:18, where Jesus refers to the fruit of the vine. That word is *genëmatos.*

RICH IN VITAMINS, MINERALS, FIBER, AND ENZYMES

Fresh fruits and vegetables are rich in:

- *Vitamins* that help regulate metabolism—converting fat and carbohydrates into energy and assisting in forming bone and tissues.
- *Minerals* that are important in maintaining physiological processes, strengthening skeletal structures, and preserving the vigor of the heart and the brain as well as all muscle and nerve systems.
- *Fiber* that is important for keeping the body cleansed and free from the problem of constipation.
- *Enzymes*—the active materials in the digestive juices that cause the chemical breakdown of food for assimilation.[2]

Examples of fruit nutritional claims:
- *Grapes* are rich in iron and potassium and are acclaimed as a strong cleansing agent.
- *Lemons* contain vitamin C, calcium, phosphorus, and magnesium. They are also acclaimed as an antiseptic, a preventive of disease, and an excellent cleanser of impurities in the system. (Lemon juice is also an excellent gargle for a sore throat).[3]
- *Papayas* contain an enzyme called papain that acts on starches and emulsifies fats and is a tremendous aid to digestion. Because it also breaks down protein, this enzyme is used as a meat tenderizer and in medicine. Papayas are a good source of fiber and folate and are rich in vitamins C and A. (Vitamin A is rare in fruits.)
- *Oranges* are one of nature's finest gifts. They are rich in salts, especially lime and alkaline salts, that counteract the tendency to acidosis. Orange juice is especially suited in time of fever to help relieve and quench the fever's fire and eliminate poison through the skin and kidneys.

- *Apples* are a great source of vitamins and much-needed fiber for our daily diet. One apple has 20 percent of the fiber our bodies need each day. About 80 percent of the fiber found in apples is soluble, while the rest is insoluble. Soluble fiber can help lower blood cholesterol and insoluble fiber may prevent certain types of cancer. Fresh apple juice made from unpeeled apples is rich in vitamins A, B₁, B₆, C, biotin, folic acid, plus much more!

Examples of vegetable nutritional claims:

- *Broccoli* is often called the "Crown Jewel of Nutrition" because it is loaded with vitamins, high in fiber, and low in calories. A medium size stalk of broccoli provides 220 percent of your daily value of vitamin C.
- *Celery* is considered the second most important salad crop in America. Two medium stalks have only 20 calories and provide 15 percent of the vitamin C your body needs every day. Plus, they are loaded with fiber and potassium.
- *Potatoes* are a good source of vitamin C, potassium, and fiber—just one serving of potatoes has 12 percent of the fiber we need every day. And it's best to eat them with the skins on! Potato skins contain fiber, potassium, iron, calcium, zinc, phosphorus, and B vitamins.
- *Carrots* are a great source of vitamin A. Have you ever wondered what makes carrots orange? Beta-carotene. Our bodies convert beta-carotene into vitamin A. One carrot has 220 percent of the vitamin A we need every day! Carrots are also a source of fiber, potassium, and vitamin C.
- *Asparagus* is rich in a B vitamin called folacin, which contributes to the duplication of cells for growth and repair of the body and blood cell reproduction in the bone marrow. It also contains glutathione, which is one of the body's most potent cancer fighters. And asparagus is high in rutin, which is valuable in strengthening the blood vessels.

I strive to eat at least one large raw vegetable salad every day. I store the following in a large container each week: romaine lettuce, red leaf lettuce, and spinach. I cut up the other ingredients such as tomatoes, cucumbers, green peppers, broccoli, cauliflower, onions, carrots, mushrooms, black olives, radishes, and avocados.

HEALTH-GIVING SUBSTANCES

The health-giving benefits of fruits and vegetables have been emphasized for many years in the health food world. But recently the claims for these good foods have even made it into popular magazines and other media.

Ongoing research is being performed to examine the effect of diet on a number of metabolic diseases such as cancer, diabetes, arthritis, gall bladder disease, osteoporosis, diverticulitis, and others. "The National Cancer Institute says that about one-third of all cancers are linked to diet; other experts put the figure as high as 60 percent. The most recent research provides consistent findings that what we eat may prevent some of the most widespread cancers, including those of breast, lungs, and colon, as well as the most intractable, such as pancreatic."[4]

Top Cancer-Fighting Foods

- *Yellow, Orange, and Red Vegetables and Fruits* (rich in beta-carotene). One of the main cancer-fighting substances is beta-carotene. It is found in deep green and brightly colored yellow, orange, and red vegetables such as carrots, sweet potatoes, and pumpkins. Fruits high in beta-carotene include apricots and cantaloupes.

- *Red Fruits and Vegetables* (rich in lycopene). Tomatoes have the highest concentrations of lycopene, a substance more powerful even than beta-carotene in attacking certain toxins that can trigger cancer in cells. The compound is also found in watermelon and red peppers.

- *Green Leafy Vegetables* (rich in antioxidants). An Italian study indicates that dark green leafy vegetables can lower the risk of many cancers. Vegetables such as spinach, kale, broccoli, and dark green lettuces are full of antioxidants, beta-carotene, and folate, as well as lutein. The darker the vegetable's color, the higher in antioxidants it is.

- *Garlic and Onions.* More than thirty cancer-fighting chemicals have been identified in garlic, onions, and even scallions. A study at Penn State University showed that feeding rats fresh garlic blocked 70 percent of breast tumors. In humans, studies show that those who eat more onions and garlic are less prone to stomach cancer.[5]

- *Cruciferous Vegetables.* One reason Asians may have lower cancer rates than Westerners is that Asian diets include more cruciferous vegetables such as cabbage and bok choy. Certain anti-cancer compounds called indoles are also found in cauliflower, broccoli, brussels sprouts, kale, mustard greens, and turnips. It is best to eat these vegetables raw or lightly cooked, as heavy cooking may destroy the anti-cancer compounds.

- *Soy Products.* Studies suggest that people who frequently consume soy foods have a lower cancer rate. A 1995 study published in the *New England Journal of Medicine* found that replacing meat with soy protein cut cholesterol levels by an average of 10 percent and dangerously high cholesterol levels by 20 percent in only a month's time.

BRING ON MORE FRUITS AND VEGETABLES

A review of 170 studies from seventeen nations pointed out that people who eat the most fruits and vegetables have half the cancer rates of those who eat the least. That includes cancers of the lung, colon, breast, cervix, esophagus, stomach, bladder, pancreas, and ovaries.

When and how you eat fruits and vegetables is also important. The fresher, the better, but even dried fruits and vegetables have many good nutrients left. When appropriate, eat fruits and vegetables with the skins. Dr. Rex Russell in *What the Bible Says About Healthy Living* says:

> The longer the storage time, the greater the loss of nutrients . . .
> the fresher they are, the better. Vitamin C is lost the quickest, but
> many other important nutrients remain. . . . A rating of the most
> nourishing forms of fruits and vegetables, including ways to prepare them, looks like this: (1) raw, (2) steamed, (3) baked, (4) soups
> or broth, (5) freshly squeezed juice, (6) frozen, (7) stir-fried, (8)
> canned . . . (25!) deep-fried.[6]

The National Cancer Institute says to strive for five or more servings of fruits and vegetables a day. I encourage you to try to eat one citrus fruit a day and one apple a day, plus other types of fruit in season. I always keep a large bowl of fresh fruit on my kitchen counter at all times. I keep grapes in a separate bowl to encourage "pick-up" snacks instead of chips or cookies.

Are you getting your five a day? The following guidelines have been established to determine one serving of fruits and vegetables:

- one medium fruit or ½ cup of small or chopped fruit
- ¾ cup (6 oz.) of 100 percent juice
- ¼ cup dried fruit
- ½ cup raw non-leafy or cooked vegetables
- one cup raw leafy vegetables (such as lettuce)
- ½ cup cooked beans or peas (such as lentils, pinto beans, and kidney beans)[7]

WHAT ABOUT VITAMIN AND MINERAL SUPPLEMENTS?

Just about anywhere you do your shopping—even in the mall—you'll find an outlet for vitamin and mineral supplements. Why? Because America is gorging on foods that contain empty calories! And much of what we eat from the garden is grown in soil that has been stripped of many of its nutrients. For these reasons, I take supplements each day.

There are many opinions on vitamin and mineral supplements. Research shows that taking supplements of vitamins E, C, and B complex, beta-carotene, and others can help, but they can never replace the nutrient value you get from eating food. This is why we need to eat healthful food and supplement daily to make sure our bodies are getting what they need.

One supplement that is popular is a product manufactured from the juice of young barley leaves. It is available in powder and tablet form and provides many nutrients and enzymes. You simply take it daily with your favorite juice, as recommended. To find out more about this supplement and more, I encourage you to stop by your local health food store and review the many resource materials available. Also I encourage you to consult with your doctor or pharmacist to see which supplements are best for you, because some can interact with prescription medicines.

A book that contains valuable information about vitamins, minerals, and food supplements is *Prescription for Nutritional Healing* by James F. Balch, M.D. and Phyllis A. Balch, C.N.C.

WHY NOT TRY JUICING?

Hardly anyone eats enough vegetables, so why not try juicing for greater nutrition and energy? Juicing is a great way to get more nutritional value from vegetables. Canned, bottled, or frozen juices just cannot match the flavor and food value of freshly squeezed juices.

And if you want to get the most when you juice, make sure you use vegetables as your main ingredients. They are the most valuable. Green veggies are very good to juice, but they need something more to help the taste. Carrots make a perfect base for juicing. They're good and good for you. They also bring out the flavor of other fruits and vegetables when blended together.

Some delicious juices can be made with carrots, cucumbers, and celery. For a refreshing change, throw in a Granny Smith apple and some lemon juice! Add half a beet to your carrot juice for a delicious and very nutritious drink. Or add some green pepper, cabbage, or spinach to your carrot juice. Just about anything that is grown in the vegetable garden can be juiced!

Fruit, on the other hand, is more easily eaten whole, and too much fruit juice is high in sugar content and calories. Although some fruit juices are certainly good, they shouldn't be consumed instead of or in the same way as water.

If you think juicing is something you'd like to begin doing, you can purchase a juicer and/or buy a book on juicing at your local health food store (basic recipes usually come with your juicer). Just remember, juice only as much as you'll drink immediately. Much of the nutritional value is lost after twenty minutes. I use juicing as preventative medicine. My goal is one big glass of fresh vegetable juice a day.

NUTRITIONAL CLAIMS FOR THE GRAPE

Grapes have become famous on account of the publicity given to the "grape cure" for cancer. Although grapes are low in vitamins, they are great cleansers of the body. They are useful in cases of anemia, low blood pressure, sluggish liver, catarrhal conditions, obesity, and skin trouble. However, they should not be used in cases of inflammation of the digestive tract or diabetes.[8]

"The reason grapes get the results they do is because they have great dissolving qualities, and their valuable iron content helps to build up the blood. However, if the poisons are dissolved without being eliminated, trouble results. So it is much better to use carrot juice and distilled water for a time before attempting the 'grape cure.'" Carrot juice not only heals, but it contains most of the minerals and vitamins to build good healthy cells and tissues. Grapes are the food third highest in iron. They are numbered among the principal foods for carbon. Some grapes contain calcium; some contain a trace of iodine. Grapes from some rocky countries contain boron. Green grapes are good for the complexion because they contain arsenic. Grapes yield an alkaline ash, found between the skin and fiber in the fruit. This ash neutralizes toxic conditions in the body—hence the reason for chewing and swallowing the grape skin.[9] (Frederick W. Collins, who consulted with many of the food laboratories in the world and the Food and Drug Adminstration, worked out the analysis of the grape.)

Grape Juice—Protection Against Heart Attack?

"Thus says the LORD: 'As the new wine [*tiyrowsh*: grape juice] is found in the cluster, and one says, "Do not destroy it, for a blessing is in it . . ."'" (Isaiah 65:8a). For years researchers have espoused the benefits of drinking wine as a preventative measure against heart attack. More recently though studies have determined that the alcohol content in red wine is not the factor primarily responsible for reducing cardiovascular disease (CVD).

Instead, researchers from all over the world are discovering that antioxidants, called *flavonoids*, are the protective agents helping fight CVD. And where can you find these helpful flavonoids? Apples, onions, broccoli, and, for our particular interest in this section, purple grapes.

From the University of Florida, Patrick J. Bird, Ph.D., says:

Plants manufacture some 1,000 different flavonoids. But one—resveratrol—from the skin of the red grapes, seems to be most effective in the battle against heart disease. Resveratrol acts by decreasing the stickiness of blood cells that aid in clotting. . . . Grapes are the richest source of resveratrol. . . . Besides offering some protection against heart disease, it has been shown to decrease the activity of free-radical reactions that are linked to several cancers.[10]

In November 1998, the American Heart Association released this good news: "Purple grape juice seems to have the same effect as red wine in reducing the risk of heart disease."[11] Jane E. Freedman, M.D., assistant professor of medicine and pharmacology at Georgetown University Medical Center, Washington, D.C., studied the blood platelets (blood cells that clump to form blood clots) in controlled solutions of grape juice. She states, "A platelet has to be activated to form blood clots. The study showed that this flavonoid [quercetin] inhibits platelets, which may explain the beneficial effect of purple grape products in heart disease."[12]

Other researchers have joined the chorus singing the praises of the grape. Researchers from the University of Wisconsin reported in the journal *Circulation* that grape juice helps the blood flow more freely. Building upon past research, this study suggests that the flavonoids (antioxidant compounds) found in the grape are in part responsible for this good news.[13]

In defense of the grape over wine, one researcher, John Folts, Ph.D., at the University of Wisconsin had this to say:

> Wine only prevents blood from clotting (when it's consumed) at levels high enough to declare someone legally drunk. With grape juice, you can drink enough to get the benefit without worrying about becoming intoxicated. What's more, alcoholic drinks don't seem to improve the function of cells in blood vessel linings the way grape juice does. And alcohol generates free radicals—unstable oxygen molecules that can actually cause damage to blood vessel tissues—dampening any of the benefits that red wine's antioxidants may offer.[14]

In further research, wine has been shown to increase levels of HDL, the "good" cholesterol, in the blood. However, because of the health hazards of intoxicating wine (i.e., liver damage), it is best to avoid wine and increase your HDLs some other way.

Theologian Dr. Charles Wesley Ewing comments on the effects of wine:

Any beverage that contains alcohol contains poison. Fermented wine contains alcohol, a poison, an intoxicant, a hypnotic, an analgesic, an anesthetic, and a potentially habit-forming, craving-producing, addiction-producing drug. To this writer, it is inconceivable that an all-wise God, with the best interests of His creatures in mind, would give His sanction to the use of any drink that contains poison, or that is an addiction-producing drug.[15]

Having said all this, I conclude that the best way to get the health benefits of the grape is to choose purple grape juice that typically contains the whole grape, including the seed. If you eat whole grapes, do what I have done for over twenty years—eat the seeds. Then you can gain the benefit of the health-giving flavonoids.

SPIRITUAL APPLICATION

The Fruit of the Vine

The juice of the grape was chosen by God to symbolize the blood of Jesus Christ. When Jesus sat with His disciples at the Last Supper, He passed a cup filled with the "fruit of the vine" saying, "This cup is the new covenant in My blood. This do, as often as you drink it, in remembrance of Me" (1 Corinthians 11:25b).

The Greek word for the "fruit of the vine" is *genëmatos* (see Matthew 26:29; Mark 14:25; 22:18). It is the word from which we get "generation" and pertains to producing or bringing forth. Grapes are a life-giving form of fruit. Leviticus 17:14 tells us that blood is the life of all flesh. On the cross Jesus willingly poured out His blood, His very life for you and me.

The Cleansing Agent of the Soul

What can wash away my sin? Nothing but the blood of Jesus.
What can make me whole again? Nothing but the blood of Jesus.
Oh, precious is the flow that makes me white as snow!
No other fount I know, nothing but the blood of Jesus.
—ROBERT LOWRY

Some nutritionists claim that the grape and grape juice are cleansing agents of the blood. If so, they would aid in the prevention and healing of diseases that flow through the blood. Is it then a coincidence or God's plan that the same element that represents the blood of Christ, which cleanses us spiritually from sin, can also be a cleansing agent of the physical blood, which keeps us free from disease? You will have to study and decide this for yourself.

Daniel Purposed in His Heart

> But Daniel purposed in his heart that he would not defile himself with the portion of the king's delicacies, nor with the wine which he drank; therefore he requested of the chief of the eunuchs that he might not defile himself. (Daniel 1:8)

Daniel made a creative request. He asked the king's servant to give him and his friends a diet of only vegetables to eat and water to drink for ten days (read the full account in Daniel 1). At the end of the ten days, Daniel and his friends were healthier looking than those who ate the king's delicacies.

God honored this commitment by bringing the Israelite captives into the favor and good will of their overseer. God also blessed them with wisdom and knowledge ten times greater than that possessed by all the magicians and astrologers. I know that God honors this kind of commitment, even today.

Besides the benefits of good health that came to Daniel and his friends from this wise choice, we discover a deeper spiritual principle. That principle is: "He who is faithful in what is least is faithful also in much; and he who is unjust in what is least is unjust also in much" (Luke 16:10).

God allows us to be tested in the more mundane matters of life to see if we can be trusted. Lamentations 3:27-28 says, "It is good for a man to bear the yoke in his youth. Let him sit alone and keep silent, because God has laid it on him." Those who do not pass the tests of discipline in youth cannot be trusted in places of greater responsibility in later years.

Daniel was promoted because he was found faithful in even the small things. He could also be counted on to be faithful in that which was much. Our faithfulness may not always win a promotion.

Remember when Daniel's prayerful faithfulness to God landed him in the lion's den! But guess who intervened? Right! God Himself shut the mouths of the lions.

I hope this chapter has caused you to take a closer look not only into your food pantry, but also into your heart. Psalm 119:9 asks each of us, "How can a young man cleanse his way?" Then it answers, "By taking heed according to Your Word." May you hide His Word in your heart and keep yourself pure for the work He wants to do through you.

ASK YOURSELF

In a practical sense, "Am I the master of my appetite—making hard choices every day to make sure my body gets what it needs—not necessarily what it wants? When I eat out, am I carried away by the delicacies of this world and find it hard to make wise choices about what's healthy for me? At the grocery store, do the dessert aisles look more appealing than the produce area? When was the last time I chose a cluster of purple grapes (with the seeds) or a glass of grape juice for dessert? Which is better for me—preparing a salad from scratch or warming up a frozen dinner in the microwave?"

Let the Holy Spirit move inside your heart as you ask, "Am I trusting in the blood of Christ to cleanse me from all sin? Am I abiding in the Vine each and every day to get the nourishment and sustenance I need to grow strong as a child of God? When was the last time I purposed in my heart to obey God in the area of eating? If someone followed me around for one week, or even a day, what would they discover about my faithfulness in the small things?"

A Bright Idea for Healthy Eating . . .

If I could get you to start practicing one good idea today, it would be for you to begin eating purple grapes (the whole grape) on a regular basis. Buy a nice, big juicy cluster and enjoy!

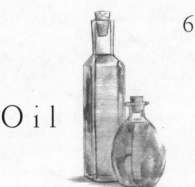

Oil

. . . a land of olive oil . . .

DEUTERONOMY 8:8

A LAND OF OLIVE OIL

The Bible provides much instruction on how to maintain good health. A part of that plan is for us to have the right balance of grains, dairy and meat products, fruits and vegetables, and oils in our daily diets. But where do we draw the line on how much and what kind of oils and/or fats to eat?

First let's draw the line between fats and oils. Oils and fats are both mentioned in the Old Testament, but only oil is mentioned in the New Testament. The Hebrew word *shemen* and the Greek word *elaion* are the words most often used for oil in the Old and New Testaments, respectively, and they refer to the oil from olives.

Shemen was used for lighting, anointing, and burning (see Exodus 25:6; 35:28). It was also used for cooking purposes (see Numbers 11:8; Deuteronomy 8:8). In the New Testament *elaion* was primarily used for lighting and anointing (see Matthew 25:3-4; Mark 6:13; Luke 7:46; Hebrews 1:9; James 5:14).

Now fat is another issue altogether. When the Bible talks about fat, it is typically referring to fats used for sacrifices and eating. For instance, Leviticus 3:17 says, "This shall be a perpetual statute throughout your generations in all your dwellings: you shall eat neither fat nor blood." What kind of fat is this? In his enlightening book, *What the*

Bible Says About Healthy Living, Dr. Rex Russell writes: "When Leviticus 3:17 forbids eating fat, it is not referring to the internal, marbling fat in the meat of clean animals, but to two other kinds of fat: the fat of unclean animals and the cover fat, including that of clean animals."[1]

Even modern nutritional advice tells us to avoid eating the "cover fat" that is next to the skin of the animal. Dr. Russell raises another important issue in talking about fats, and that is: What are unclean and clean animals? What does the Bible—the New and Old Testament—say about eating meat? Are we to eat only the clean animals discussed in the Old Testament, or does the "new law" of the New Testament give us more liberty? Stay tuned for the next chapter on meats. For now, let's move on.

GOOD FAT OR BAD FAT?

In the 1930s and 1940s the so-called experts, using the knowledge of the time, declared that "eating fat is good for you." During the next fifty years they changed their tune to "fat is bad." Fats labeled bad in the 1960s through the 1980s included butter, avocados, grains, nuts, olives, and their oil.

How do we decide which fats are good and which ones are bad? Certainly, there is a lot of confusion for those of us concerned about good health.

The first place I turned to for answers was the Bible. You've already read much of what I discovered in God's Word about the difference between fats and oils (and you'll read more at the conclusion of this chapter). The rest I discovered by reading about the molecular structure of fats and oils and how they can benefit or harm our bodies.

In his book *Fats That Kill, Fats That Heal,* Udo Erasmus says, "The fact is that some fats are absolutely required for health, while others are detrimental. Whether a fat heals or kills depends on several factors: What kind of fat is it?

- How has it been treated—is it fresh; has it been exposed to light, oxygen, heat, hydrogen, water, acid, base, or metals like copper and iron?
- How old is it?
- How has it been used in food preparation?

- How much was eaten?
- What balance of different fats do we get?"[2]

Saturated vs. Unsaturated: What's the Difference?

What is fat saturated with in order to be called a saturated fat? Our government's Consumer Information Center provides the answer: "There are three main types of fatty acids: saturated, monounsaturated and polyunsaturated. All fatty acids are molecules composed mostly of carbon and hydrogen atoms. A saturated fatty acid has the maximum possible number of hydrogen atoms attached to every carbon atom. It is therefore said to be 'saturated' with hydrogen atoms."[3]

The Good Fats—Unsaturated

Essential Fatty Acids. EFAs are probably the most important and least understood of all the fats. The major building blocks of all fats, they are eventually converted into important compounds called prostaglandins (PGs). PGs are necessary for many physiological functions, including inflammatory response, energy production, tissue growth and repair, blood pressure regulation, and fat metabolism.

The body must have a constant supply of EFAs, but most people do not eat enough EFA-rich foods (certain nuts, seeds, oils, and cold-water fish) to meet their nutritional needs. An inadequate intake of EFAs and an overconsumption of "bad" fats increases the risk of developing disease.[4]

Polyunsaturated Fatty Acids. PFAs are necessary for organ and glandular function. They are extremely fluid because of their chemical nature. They remain liquid at room temperature, in the refrigerator, and most importantly in the body where they are needed to keep cell membranes fluid and flexible. Usually these fats come from vegetables, seeds, nuts, and fish.

These fatty acids can neutralize the negative effects of saturated fats if the polyunsaturates outnumber the saturates. Omega-3 polyunsaturated fatty acids are found in fish, such as salmon and mackerel, as well as in soybean, canola, and flaxseed oil and in walnuts. Some research has shown that these acids lower both the LDL cholesterol and triglyceride levels in the blood.[5]

Monounsaturated Fatty Acids. MFAs have a different chemical structure than polyunsaturated fats. They remain liquid at room and body temperature, but they solidify in the refrigerator. MFAs tend to lower blood cholesterol, especially when used to replace saturated fatty acids.

You can find this type of fat in olive, canola, and peanut oil, as well as in meats, nuts, and seeds. Oleic acid, found in olive, avocado, and peanut oils, is probably the most important monounsaturated fatty acid because it helps keep arteries supple.

The Bad Fats—Saturated and Hydrogenated

Saturated Fatty Acids. SFAs are used primarily for energy and insulation and usually are found in meat from land animals. Most people get all the saturated fat they need from their regular diet of carbohydrates, proteins, and other unsaturated fats, so there is no need for them to eat more saturated fats.

Not only that, but saturated fats can be harmful. They are not fluid, and they remain solid in the body. Thus they have a tendency to stick together and form clots after they're ingested. Eating too many saturated fats increases your risk of cardiovascular disease—one of the leading causes of death in this country.

Hydrogenated and Trans-Fatty Acids. These fatty acids are unsaturated oils that have undergone a process in which they are converted to a solid form of fat. The hydrogenation process was introduced by Proctor and Gamble in 1911 with their first commercially hydrogenated shortening called Crisco. The company had two goals in mind when they introduced this product. One was to produce an inexpensive, spreadable product such as margarine, and the second was to handle the problem of unsaturated fats spoiling too quickly. In other words— longer shelf life! Unfortunately, shortening promotes shorter human life! Corporate America was not interested in your health.

These fats result in clogged arteries and high blood pressure, and they're found in vegetable shortening, margarine, most peanut butter (unless the oil is still at the top), cookies, breads, crackers, and commercial bakery products.[6]

THE OIL OF THE OLIVE

God brought the children of Israel into a good land that contained olive oil (see Deuteronomy 8:8). And throughout Scripture we read that olive oil was used in cooking, anointing, lighting, and sacrificing. God knew what He was creating and prescribing for His children.

We know today that olive oil is very healthy. "It contains anti-cancer properties, leads to more efficient cardiac contractions, and does not lead to vascular disease. At Johns Hopkins University, studies have shown that olive oil is digested in a process similar to complex carbohydrates."[7] Olive oil was the choice of our biblical ancestors and should be our choice today!

Other vegetable oils such as flaxseed, sunflower, safflower, and canola oils are also healthful. But when any of these "good" oils are hydrogenated, they become bad for you. "The hydrogenation of these oils saturates them and makes them solid. They then actually become toxic when their structures are changed."[8]

BUTTER VERSUS MARGARINE

The whole controversy over butter and margarine started years ago when margarine was highly publicized because it had no cholesterol and was high in polyunsaturated oils. Is butter really as bad as some people say it is? Let's examine the molecular structure and health benefits of each to decide.

> Butter is basically a natural product, and its fatty acids are structurally similar to the fatty acids in our bodies. The heat and chemicals used to transform vegetable oils into margarine change fatty acids into unnatural forms that may be harmful to our health.
>
> Unsaturated fatty acids have points of molecular strain where carbon atoms are connected to each other by double or triple bonds instead of being fully occupied by hydrogen atoms. These strain points determine the three-dimensional configurations of molecules.
>
> In nature all of these molecules have a curved shape that allows them to fit neatly into the membranes that enclose all cells and many of the structures within them. Chemists call this natural shape the *cis*-configuration. Heat and harsh chemical treatment can cause unsaturated fatty acids to spring open into a different shape called the *trans*-configuration, which looks jointed instead of curved.
>
> The body cannot incorporate trans-fatty acids into its membranes, and if it tries to do so, deformed cellular structures may result. Eating trans-fatty acids in margarine, vegetable shorten-

ing, and partially hydrogenated vegetable oils probably increases cancer risk, promotes inflammation, and accelerates aging and degenerative changes in tissues.[9]

We read about butter in the first part of Deuteronomy 32:14 (KJV): "Butter of kine [from the cattle], and milk of the flock." This passage refers to all the good things that God had given His people for their good. The Bible is clearly saying that butter is good. Therefore eat butter instead of margarine, but do so sparingly.

TOO MUCH FAT

For years health organizations have advised us against eating too much fat. The American Heart Association tells us that heart diseases, strokes, and other related disorders kill almost as many people as all other causes of death combined. Arteriosclerosis (a buildup of fatty deposits within artery walls that restricts and sometimes blocks blood to the vital organs) is the main culprit.

A WORD ON CHOLESTEROL

James and Phyllis Balch write extensively on the subject of cholesterol in their book *Prescription for Nutritional Healing*:

> Elevated blood cholesterol and triglyceride levels lead to plaque-filled arteries, with impeded blood flow to the brain, kidney, genitals, extremities, and heart. High cholesterol is a primary cause for heart disease because it produces fatty deposits in the arteries. Other conditions that are implicated by high cholesterol levels are gallstones, impotence, mental impairment, and high blood pressure. Colon polyps and cancer (especially prostrate and breast cancer) have also been linked to high cholesterol levels.[10]

There are two kinds of cholesterol: LDL (the unwanted type) and HDL (the beneficial type). The total cholesterol number is not as important as the individual LDL and HDL numbers. The HDL number, of course, should be the highest number.

To increase HDL, the polyunsaturated fats must outnumber the saturates. However, too much fat of any kind adds too many calories and has an adverse effect on the body. Here is a statistic to note:

The daily food intake of Americans in general is 40 percent fats. This should be cut 25 to 30 percent or less.

"If we get the right kinds of fats in the right amounts and balances, and prepare them using the right methods, they build our health. The wrong kinds of fats, the wrong amounts or balances, or even the right kinds of fats wrongly prepared cause degenerative diseases."[11]

Diet greatly affects cholesterol levels. If you struggle with keeping your cholesterol level in a healthy range, then you need to recognize that foods high in saturated fats (especially animal fat) will drive up your unwanted LDLs. However, a diet rich in vegetables (especially raw green, red, and yellow vegetables) and fruits can lower cholesterol.

Although this section is about the effect of different kinds of fats on your cholesterol, it needs to be noted that exercise and niacin are two chief contributors to help increase the good HDLs.

THE NO-FAT MYTH

Many people are getting on the no-fat bandwagon. Sounds like a good idea, doesn't it? It is true that fats in large quantities are harmful. However, some fat is good, so don't "throw the baby out with the bathwater."

Also let me tell you something that you won't hear from the makers of "no-fat" and "low-fat" products. Just because something is "low-fat" or "no-fat" doesn't mean you can eat all you want. This is a great myth and an even greater deception. Many "no-fat" and "low-fat" foods are laden with sugar and other high-calorie, no-food-value ingredients. Worse yet, these ingredients eventually turn into fat in your body.

Yes, we need to start with a basic knowledge of fat grams. Next we shouldn't eat too many fats. But let's be sensible! Read those labels! Study the caloric value, as well as the ingredients and the serving size. You'll be surprised by how easily you can be fooled by the manufacturer.

SPIRITUAL APPLICATION

Oil in My Lamp

When I was a teenager, we sang a chorus titled "Give Me Oil in My Lamp." It concluded, "Keep me burning till the break of day." That oil in the lamp was a symbol of the Holy Spirit. Without His continual filling, we would spiritually burn out because we would be just burn-ing the wick and not drawing from Him.

When my youngest daughter Janice was about ten years old, a godly Bible teacher from England, Major Ian Thomas, spoke at our church. Each time he entered the pulpit, he would teach for about an hour. As you might expect, this became quite lengthy for my ten-year-old. One day after a service, she was "complaining" about how long it had been. She said, "He just went on and on about gas in the car, oil in the lamp, and God in the man."

I was quite amused. For even though it may have been long for a lit-tle girl, she had certainly gotten the message. Major Thomas had effec-tively used those illustrations to show the importance of the Holy Spirit's continual filling in our lives.

The lamp stand in the Old Testament temple was always kept burn-ing. There had to be a constant supply of oil. This is an illustration of our dependence upon the Holy Spirit to keep our lives aflame with passion and power.

In the New Testament we read about another aspect of that oil that needs to keep burning brightly for God. Jesus tells this parable about the ten virgins:

> *Then the kingdom of heaven shall be likened to ten virgins who took their lamps and went out to meet the bridegroom. Now five of them were wise, and five were foolish. Those who were foolish took their lamps and took no oil with them, but the wise took oil in their vessels with their lamps. But while the bridegroom was delayed, they all slumbered and slept.*

> *And at midnight a cry was heard: "Behold, the bridegroom is com-ing; go out to meet him!" Then all those virgins arose and trimmed their lamps. And the foolish said to the wise, "Give us some of your oil, for our lamps are going out." But the wise answered, saying, "No, lest there should not be enough for us and you; but go rather to those who sell, and buy for yourselves."*

> *And while they went to buy, the bridegroom came, and those who were ready went in with him to the wedding; and the door was shut. Afterward the other virgins came also, saying, "Lord, Lord, open to us!" But he answered and said, "Assuredly, I say to you, I do not*

know you." Watch therefore, for you know neither the day nor the
hour in which the Son of Man is coming. (Matthew 25:1-13)

Yes, Lord, give me oil in my lamp. Keep me burning! Keep me burning till the break of day. I hope you will be like the wise bride who had her oil lamp lit and ready when the bridegroom came to claim her as His bride. Take some time today to fill your lamp with His oil of hope, joy, and contentment.

ASK YOURSELF

Now ask yourself, "Have I jumped on the 'low-fat' or 'no-fat' bandwagon without considering that in giving up fat, I may be consuming extra calories that will eventually turn into fat? Am I choosing the right amount of good fats in my daily diet? How do I prepare my meals? Do I play the 'dash-and-trash' game at the fast-food chains? Or do I make mealtime a sit-down occasion with healthy choices for me and my family?"

Examine your walk with Jesus by asking, "What am I filling up with to keep me burning brightly for Jesus? Am I filling up with people, possessions, or position? Or am I filling myself up with the person of Jesus Christ? Is the Holy Spirit's oil of gladness in my heart and flowing out to others? Have I let my light go out because I was pursuing other things? Or am I seeking Him with all my heart as a bride awaiting her bridegroom?"

A Bright Idea for Healthy Eating . . .

You can now spray your way to healthy eating! Try the new sprays of olive oil and butter for "buttering" your cookware and skillets. I also recommend spraying a little on your veggies for a buttery flavor!

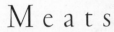

Meats

*And when
your herds and
your flocks multiply . . .*

DEUTERONOMY 8:13

*Every moving thing that lives
shall be food for you.*

GENESIS 9:3

GOD'S PROVISION

Herds and flocks are mentioned in Deuteronomy 8:13 as part of God's
provision in His good land. However, the first time that meat is mentioned in the Bible as food is in Genesis 9:3-4 when God said to Noah,
"Every moving thing that lives shall be food for you. I have given you
all things, even as the green herbs. But you shall not eat flesh with its life,
that is, its blood."

Another Old Testament reference to eating meat concerns Jacob
preparing "savory meat" for his father Isaac in Genesis 27:9. Also the
eating of the Passover lamb was an integral part of the exodus from
Egypt. Then, of course, the killing and eating of the Passover lamb
continued from Old Testament times into the days of the New

Testament, when Jesus ate the Passover with His disciples. The Feast of the Passover is celebrated by the Jewish people to this day.

When the prodigal son came home, the father instructed the servants to "kill the fatted calf," and feasting and rejoicing followed (see Luke 15:11-32). Jesus multiplied the loaves and fishes and fed the multitudes (see Matthew 14:15-21). Jesus also cooked fish for the disciples after His resurrection at the Sea of Galilee (see Luke 24:41-43 and John 21:9-13).

The Bible clearly states God's provision of meat for food and His blessing on it in general. He did, however, give some specific instructions about what meat to eat and how it is to be prepared. There are differences of opinion about some of the interpretations of Scripture concerning these matters. One should study these issues to determine for oneself what is best.

This chapter on meat is somewhat longer than the other chapters, for this subject is sometimes controversial and may be perplexing to some. The Bible has some clarifying insights that I would like to share with you.

Old Testament Insights

Dr. J. Sidlow Baxter, a well-known preacher, author, and Bible teacher, has much to say about the dietary law of the Old Testament. In his book *Our High Calling*, he has a chapter titled "Sanctification and the Dietary Law." He writes:

> Included in the "judgments" or "statutes" of the Mosaic Law there is what may be described as the dietary code. Whenever we read it, we should always say to ourselves, "This is God speaking." If anyone knows what is proper for the body, He who made it does. I believe that many of our race's bodily ills would begin at once to disappear if we observed merely the main proscriptions of the Mosaic dietary guide.[1]

The Old Testament dietary law found in Leviticus 11 and Deuteronomy 14 gives a list of clean animals that God gave as "good" meat to be eaten and a list of unclean animals that God said should not be eaten.

Most evangelical Christians have considered the dietary law part of the ceremonial law and therefore not applicable to them. However, I have studied this issue and believe that the ceremonial law and the dietary law were two different entities. I believe the ceremonial law was fulfilled in Jesus Christ. And I believe the dietary law has many commonsense applications today.

I encourage you to study this issue for yourself, since I am not able to adequately address this vast area of biblical doctrine in the scope of this book. Two good books on this subject are *God's Key to Health and Happiness* by Elmer Josephson and *What the Bible Says About Healthy Living* by Rex Russell, M.D.

For now, let me summarize by giving two verses from the book of Leviticus regarding clean and unclean animals. The Lord gave Moses and Aaron guidelines for eating animals. Concerning those animals that lived on land: "Among the animals, whatever divides the hoof, having cloven hooves and chewing the cud—that you may eat" (Leviticus 11:3).

Some of the clean animals that would be included in this list are cattle, deer, goats, oxen, sheep, geese, chickens, ducks, quails, turkeys, and a host of fish including rainbow trout, tuna, flounder, and salmon. As for unclean animals, there are only a few that we would even care to eat (i.e., rabbits, swine).

Why do Americans, and much of the world, choose to eat hogs even though they are on the list of those animals God named as unclean in the Old Testament? Bacon, ham, and sausage—all are included in many people's diets. Where would breakfast be without a slice of ham, bacon, or sausage next to a generous portion of eggs and a buttery biscuit? Hopefully, it would be on someone else's plate! Nutritionally, bacon contains a considerable amount of fat and nitrates (preservatives that have been linked to cancer). As to other unclean animals—dogs, horses, and rats—these are eaten in some parts of the world, but thankfully the prospect is repulsive to us in the West.

Concerning the animals that lived in the sea: "These you may eat of all that [are] in the water: whatever in the water has fins and scales, whether in the seas or in the rivers—that you may eat" (Leviticus 11:9). Many people enjoy eating the unclean animals on this list—shrimp, crab, lobster, oysters, snails, and catfish—all unclean according to Leviticus 11:9. (Read all of Leviticus 11 to learn the complete dietary law.)

Please note that the designations of clean and unclean animals were given before God gave the dietary law. In Genesis 7:2 God told Noah to take into the ark clean beasts by seven pairs and unclean beasts and fowls by two pairs. Now have you ever heard about the clean beasts going into the ark by seven pairs or seen a storybook or any other representation of the ark with animals and fowl going in by seven pairs? But it is written there just as plain as it can be for all to read.

New Testament Insights

Acts 10:24—11:18. One Scripture commonly used to negate the Old Testament dietary law is Peter's vision of unclean animals in Acts 10 and 11. "And a voice came to him, 'Rise, Peter; kill and eat.' But Peter said, 'Not so, Lord! For I have never eaten anything common or unclean.' And a voice spoke to him again the second time, 'What God has cleansed you must not call common'" (Acts 10:13-15).

The interpretation of the vision was clearly given—this instruction pertained to fellowshipping with Gentiles and not to eating food. Acts 10:28 says, "Then he said to them, 'You know how unlawful it is for a Jewish man to keep company with or go to one of another nation. But God has shown me that I should not call any man common or unclean.'" A sheet with unclean animals was let down from heaven. Then the sheet was again caught up into heaven. Peter never literally ate these unclean animals.

Elmer A. Josephson gives this helpful insight:

Now did the words, "Rise, Peter, kill and eat," mean that God was repealing the dietary laws? Is God reversing Himself on physical hygiene and sanitation in His requirement that a clean people have clean food? Did Christ's work on the cross perform a biological miracle in these filthy animals that made their flesh harmless to eat and fit for human consumption? Did the dispensation of grace and the coming of the Gospel so alter the gastric processes and digestive apparatus of man that all unclean meats will now build healthy bodies instead of producing disease and result in death as they did before?[2]

Indeed, the answer is no.

1 Timothy 4:1-5. Paul warns in 1 Timothy 4:3 about those who command "to abstain from foods which God created to be received with thanksgiving by those who believe and know the truth." In verse 4 he continues, "For every creature of God is good, and nothing to be refused, if it be received with thanksgiving" (KJV).

Every text needs to be seen in its context. Here God is speaking of meats that He has created to be received. There are those who were saying that it was wrong to eat even the clean food that God had created to be received. This is simply not true. Also when verse 4 says that every creature of God is good, we must conclude that God is not speaking of such things as poisonous reptiles, wild beasts, rats, cockroaches, spiders, bats, dogs, and cats. And He is certainly not approving cannibalism! We must discover truth in the light of all of God's Word.

For further insights on doubtful Scriptures, I recommend the very helpful and insightful book by Elmer A. Josephson titled *God's Key to Health and Happiness*. The author is a Baptist minister whose own serious illnesses were cured by following biblical teachings and eating natural, whole foods.

A Sign of the Last Days

That some would forbid the eating of meat that God intended for our food is one of the signs of the last days (see 1 Timothy 4:1-5). For instance, I have heard of a cult that now claims that Jesus was a vegetarian. The Bible clearly refutes this in Matthew 14:19 and John 21:12-13.

Have you noticed how animal rights groups have mushroomed since the 1960s? Read their literature and you'll discover that they are clearly going against Scripture when they say that killing and eating animals is wrong and cruel. Certainly, no one would deny that animals should be treated humanely and killed without needless suffering.

It was God who killed animals and made coats of skins to clothe Adam and Eve in the Garden of Eden (see Genesis 3:21). In mercy and compassion, He robed them in skins of animals to replace the fig-leaf aprons Adam and Eve had made. Some commentators have even used this example as an allegorical picture of Jesus—that God sent His Son to give His life and His blood to cover our sin.

As for killing animals, we have already seen that God gave permission to eat meat in Genesis 9:3 and Deuteronomy 12:15. The whole sacrificial system in the Old Testament is based on the slaying of animals. The animals that were killed and offered on the altar as sin offerings were not to be eaten. The only exceptions were the breast and the right shoulder, which were designated for the high priest and his sons to eat.

We can conclude, then, that God permits the killing and eating of animals. It is not wrong. Of course, we should never be cruel in the care of animals. Here are some verses about how God would have us treat animals: Exodus 23:5, 11; Leviticus 25:6-7; Deuteronomy 22:4, 6-7; 25:4.

Fat and Blood Forbidden

The Old Testament Proclamation. In some of the sacrificial offerings in the Old Testament, parts of the animal were to be eaten, but two elements were always forbidden as food. These were the fat and the blood: "This shall be a perpetual statute throughout your generations in all your dwellings: you shall eat neither fat nor blood" (Leviticus 3:17).

I wrote at length in the last chapter about nutrition research that has revealed the harmful effects of eating too much fat. Animal fat is especially harmful because it is totally saturated. Is this a part of God's judgment on those who eat it? We will have to judge for ourselves, because this is not clearly stated.

The spiritual reason for not eating fat is overlooked today, probably because we no longer offer animal sacrifices. The fat of the clean animal was burned on the altar as a "sweet-smelling" offering to the Lord (see Leviticus 7:31; 8:16, 25-28).

The other forbidden element is blood. The restriction against eating blood is rooted in the Old Testament and endorsed in the New Testament. God in His Word gave specific instructions on how to kill animals for sacrifice and for food. And part of the instructions banned eating the blood of the animal.

Even before the Law was given, God said, "But you shall not eat flesh with its life, that is, its *blood*" (Genesis 9:4, italics mine). This command was reiterated when the law was given. "Only be sure that you do not eat the blood, for the blood is the life; you may not eat the life with the meat. You shall not eat it; you shall pour it on the earth like water. You shall not eat it, that it may go well with you and your chil-

dren after you, when you do what is right in the sight of the LORD"
(Deuteronomy 12:23-25).

The New Testament Affirmation. The New Testament forbids the eating
of blood, as well. In Acts 15 we learn about a tolerance issue that was
ensuing between Jews and Gentiles. Amidst the heated discussion at
the Jerusalem Council, James advised the leaders to send a letter to the
Gentile Christians in Antioch, Syria, and Cilicia.

In part, this letter was to encourage the Gentile Christians to
abstain from certain practices and promote harmony between them-
selves and the Jews. Acts 15:20 gives the essence of this letter: " . . . but
that we write to them to abstain from things polluted by idols, from sexual immorality, from things strangled, and from blood."

The Spiritual and Physical Explanation. I believe there is a twofold reason for us to refrain from eating blood—physical and spiritual. Leviticus
17:14 says, " . . . for [blood] is the life of all flesh. Its blood sustains its
life." The Bible commanded that animals be slain and their blood
poured upon the earth like water (see Deuteronomy 12:16).

It was not until 1614 that man scientifically discovered that blood
is the carrier of nutrients to every part of the body. William Harvey—
the scientist behind the discovery—may have thought he was the first to
discover this truth, but God knew it all the time.

How grateful we are that the blood carries life, but how sad to discover that it also carries death. If there is disease, the blood carries that
also. If blood remains in the meat, there is a greater possibility for disease to be passed on.

Most people would be horrified at the thought of drinking or eating blood. But what they don't realize is that they're probably eating it
every time they order a steak, unless it has been properly bled.

Cattle today are not properly bled. "Cattle are stunned with a
hammer before killing, except those reserved for the kosher market.
Kosher animals are tied up, then killed by a Jewish slaughterer in a way
that ensures thorough bleeding."[3] Most of the blood is left in the
nonkosher cattle to make it weigh more and taste better.

Kosher meat is bled properly and may be purchased in the kosher
section of your grocery store or in a Jewish market. It costs more, but
your health will be worth it. If a kosher section is unavailable at your

grocery store, here are a couple of ways you can draw the blood from the meat you purchase.

- Broiling will cause much of the blood (and fat) to drip out.
- Soak the meat in water for half an hour and then spread coarse (kosher) salt on the meat. (Refined salt is too fine and will only be absorbed into the meat.) Let it set for half an hour and then rinse.

Some people are eating blood and don't even know it! And then there are some who eat meat that is known for its blood. For instance, some places in the world are known for their blood sausage. If you want to eat healthy food, eliminate the blood out of your diet.

Of all I have said on the subject, certainly the spiritual reason is the most important for not eating blood. The Old Testament says, " . . . the blood is the life" (Deuteronomy 12:23). In the New Testament we see that the blood symbolized the precious blood of Jesus and was to be held sacred:

> Not with the blood of goats and calves, but with His own blood He entered the Most Holy Place once for all, having obtained eternal redemption. For if the blood of bulls and goats and the ashes of a heifer, sprinkling the unclean, sanctifies for the purifying of the flesh, how much more shall the blood of Christ, who through the eternal Spirit offered Himself without spot to God, cleanse your conscience from dead works to serve the living God? (Hebrews 9:12-14)

IMPORTANCE OF MEAT AND PROTEIN

Now that we've discussed a little of the biblical background regarding meat, let's look at the nutritional aspects of it—most importantly, its contribution of protein to our diets. Why is it important that the body gets protein every day?

- Protein is essential for growth and development.
- Protein is a major source of building material for muscles, blood, skin, hair, nails, and internal organs, including the heart and brain.
- Protein is needed for the formation of hormones, which control growth, sexual function, and rate of metabolism.

- Protein forms enzymes necessary for basic life functions and antibodies to fight disease.[4]

Daily Protein Needs

The average person needs about 15 to 20 percent of the day's calories in protein. Find out how much protein you need by following this simple formula: Divide your ideal weight by 2.2. Now multiply that number by 0.8. The ending figure will be how many grams of protein you need to get each day.[5]

For example, if you weigh 140 pounds and your ideal weight is 120 pounds, then you need to get about 47 grams of protein each day. This translates into an ideal protein consumption of about seven ounces each day to maintain this ideal weight.

Sources of protein include meat, dairy, and vegetable products. Each has about seven to eight grams of protein per one-ounce serving. Vegetable sources of protein include legumes such as soy beans, pinto beans, black beans, kidney beans, and peas. Peanuts, walnuts, pecans, almonds, and seeds such as pumpkin, sunflower, and flaxseed are also excellent sources of protein.

If you can get protein by eating other foods, then why eat meat? Because animal foods are the best source of "complete" proteins. The protein we get from plants (soybeans are an excellent exception) is incomplete. It simply does not provide the body with all the essential amino acids.

Signs of Protein Deficiency

Typically, most Americans meet their daily protein requirement every day, so this is not an issue in the United States. But that's not the case in many other parts of the world where protein deficiencies are evidenced in malnutrition.

How do you know if you are lacking the protein needed in your daily diet? Here are some signs to look for:

- *Lack of stamina.* Is it harder for you to do the things you used to do? Do you get easily winded walking up a flight of stairs or walking from the parking lot?
- *Mental depression.* Do you feel a little blah? Think about the last two weeks or month in your life. Where would you say you

are on the "feel good" scale—1 for "really down" or 10 for "never felt better"? Or somewhere in between?

- *Poor resistance to infection.* Is it flu season and you're having a hard time fighting off the bug every time it flies by? What about that seventy-two-hour stuffy nose/headache bug that went around the office last week? Did you catch it?

- *Impaired healing of wounds.* Have you been injured lately? Take a look at the wound and see if it's healing normally or as quickly as it could. What about that paper or razor cut—how does it look today?

- *Slow recovery from disease.* Are you struggling with recovery from a disease? When you look at others who seem to bounce back, how do you compare?

Now just because you may be having these symptoms, don't jump to the conclusion that you have a protein deficiency. There could be a dozen or more reasons why you may be experiencing these things. For instance, if some of your wounds are not healing as quickly as they could, it could be a sign of diabetes. Check with your doctor and use the formula on the previous page to determine your daily protein needs.

HEALTH CONCERNS FOR MEAT EATERS

Modern science has made it possible to add growth hormones and antibiotics to the food of animals, thereby creating health problems for those who eat this meat. Health food stores and some grocery stores stock meat that does not contain these additives. You'll need to ask the butcher to make sure about this before you make a purchase.

In affluent societies such as the United States people have increased their consumption of meat over the years. Research from around the world has shown that people who eat less meat and more whole grains, fruits, and vegetables have a lower incidence of cancer and metabolic diseases.

Excess protein is stored as fat in the body tissues, so too much can make your cholesterol level soar. Too much protein can harm your kidneys and contribute to obesity and other related disorders, including osteoporosis. Your fluid l   also become imbalanced if you eat too much protein. Excessive consumption of protein in the diet or from supplements can affect the potassium levels in the system, causing heart arrhythmias.

DANGERS OF EATING PORK AND SHELLFISH

You may not know this, but the bacon you enjoy for breakfast or the ham sandwich you grab at lunch could contain more than just fat and calorie grams. It could very well have worms! And how about that steamed shellfish you enjoyed over the weekend? That may be a clambake you should have missed!

Trichinosis is a disease caused by the deadly trichina worm, one of nineteen worms found in pork. Laird S. Goldsborough writes, "In the pork, which we Americans eat, there too often lurks a myriad of baffling and sinister parasites. There are minute spiral worms called *Trichinella spilalis*. A single serving of infected pork, even a single mouthful, can kill or cripple or condemn the victim to a lifetime of aches and pains. For this unique disease, trichinosis, there is no sure cure."[6]

Senator Thomas C. Desmond, chairman of the New York Trichinosis Commission stated, "Physicians have confused trichinosis with some fifty ailments ranging from typhoid fever to alcoholism. That pain in your arm or leg may be arthritis or rheumatism, but it may be trichinosis. That pain in your back may mean a gall bladder involvement, but it may mean trichinosis."[7]

Some say that the worms will be killed with sufficient cooking, but it was reported from one lab test that trichinae-laden swine flesh was heated to an unbelievably high temperature and then put under a microscope, and some worms were still alive. Why take a chance? Do you really want to eat dead worms?

Shellfish can also cause problems. Here's a warning from the *New England Journal of Medicine* (March 13, 1986): "Increased chances of acquiring bacterial and viral diseases from raw or improperly cooked shellfish make eating these delicacies a risky venture. More than 1,000 people in New York State experienced diarrhea, nausea, vomiting, abdominal pain, cramps, and fever after eating contaminated raw oysters and clams. In addition, ten people came down with hepatitis A (infectious hepatitis)."[8]

FATTY FISH—GOOD FOR YOU

Fatty fish are good for you? Sounds like an oxymoron! But it's true. The fat in fish is not the same as the fat in animals. Fish such as salmon, mackerel, herring, and sardines are good sources of the omega-3 essential fatty acids that are so important to your health. But don't take my word for it. A British study found that people who regularly ate fish, especially fatty fish, were less likely to suffer heart attacks. In addition, a thirty-year study of 1,800 men in Illinois showed that men who consumed one or two servings of fish a week (about seven ounces) had a much lower risk of fatal heart attacks.[9]

SPIRITUAL APPLICATION

That All Would Be Well

Why did God give us the dietary law of the Old Testament? Deuteronomy 5:29b gives the answer: "That it might be well with them and with their children forever!" God didn't give us His law to burden us but to free us. My husband has said this often, and I think it applies so well:

> Have you ever thought that if you lived according to God's laws that you were going to miss out? Truth is, if you don't live according to God's law, you're going to miss out! God's laws are for your welfare. God is not a tyrant in heaven making a bunch of laws to make you squirm like a worm in hot ashes as you try to keep those laws. God loves you. Every time God says, "Thou shalt not," God is simply saying, "Don't hurt yourself." And every time God says, "Thou shalt," God is saying, "Help yourself to happiness."

Don't you want to "help yourself to happiness"? Then take God at His Word. Add the meat of His Word to your spiritual diet so you can be a strong, healthy Christian.

I pray that you will grasp the deep and abiding joy of digging deep into God's Word, meditating on its divine truth, and chewing on its golden delicacies. When you do, you'll receive the refreshment and nourishment you need to live your life as a holy vessel for His glory.

Growing Strong on the Meat of God's Word

The writer of Hebrews urges his readers to go on to maturity—to become believers who can eat strong meat. He censures them for being babies who still need to be taught the milk of the Word instead of being mature enough to be teachers: "For everyone who partakes only of milk is unskilled in the word of righteousness, for he is a babe. But solid food belongs to those who are of full age, that is, those who by reason of use have their senses exercised to discern both good and evil" (Hebrews 5:13-14).

In the next chapter the author of this letter tries to move readers beyond the foundational principles and on to the deeper issues of their faith: "*Therefore, leaving the discussion of the elementary principles of Christ, let us go on to perfection, not laying again* the foundation of repentance from dead works and of faith toward God, of the doctrine of baptisms, of laying on of hands, of resurrection of the dead, and of eternal judgment" (Hebrews 6:1-2, italics mine).

Who is a spiritual baby? One who is unskilled in the word of righteousness. Who is spiritually mature? He who has used the Word of God so often that his senses can discern both good and evil. Only by this spiritual exercise can one be mature enough to handle the strong meat of the Word.

In John 6 we read some hard sayings (strong meat) that Jesus offered the crowds that gathered around Him:

> *I am the bread of life. He who comes to Me shall never hunger, and he who believes in Me shall never thirst. (v. 35)*

> *I am the living bread which came down from heaven. If anyone eats of this bread, he will live forever; and the bread that I shall give is My flesh, which I shall give for the life of the world. (v. 51)*

> *Whoever eats My flesh and drinks My blood has eternal life, and I will raise him up at the last day. For My flesh is food indeed, and My blood is drink indeed. He who eats My flesh and drinks My blood abides in Me, and I in him. (vv. 54-56)*

Do you know what happened with this offering of strong meat? Many people didn't want it. In fact, the Word of God tells us that they quarreled and murmured about His sayings. And in the end, "many of His disciples went back and walked with Him no more" (John 6:66). May God help us to grow up—that we may be able to spiritually digest the strong meat of the Word.

ASK YOURSELF

Now ask yourself these practical questions about your eating habits: "Do I feel lethargic or full of energy—ready to face the challenges of the day? Am I eating a balanced diet? Should I cut down on the amount of meat that I am eating? When I cook chicken, do I leave the skin on? (The skin is where most of the fat is.) What change can I make in my diet today that will make a difference in how I feel and how I look— today, tomorrow, and the rest of my life?"

Yes, there are many difficult things in the Word of God. Will you give up because they are hard sayings, or will you go on to maturity through diligence and obedience? Ask yourself, "Am I still sipping on the milk, or have I moved on to learn, understand, and grow in the deeper things found in God's Word? Am I challenging myself, or am I coasting through my Christian life? Am I sitting and soaking in church, or am I allowing myself to be squeezed and poured out as His sacrificial love offering to the lost in my neighborhood, workplace, and family?"

A Bright Idea for Healthy Eating . . .

Next time you get ready to prepare meat for a meal, take time beforehand to bleed it. To do this, soak the meat in water for half an hour, then sprinkle it with kosher salt, rinse, and then broil it.

CONCLUSION

WHERE TO BEGIN

So you are convicted that you should adopt a healthier lifestyle, and you want to develop a more nutritious diet. Where should you begin?

First, you must be convinced of the necessity of changing old habits and adopting new ones. You must also be convinced of the validity of the information you've read. I can't twist your arm. In fact, no one can strong-arm you into healthy eating. It must be a decision you reach on your own through research and prayer.

Second, you must be converted. You need to have a definite change of mind and a genuine desire to turn from the old patterns and adopt a new, healthier lifestyle. If you are truly converted, you will then be changed. Some things you once loved, you will no longer desire. And some things you did not like, you will want to include in your diet now. And who knows? You may even come to like them!

Let's recap what you need to do to develop better eating habits—be convicted, be convinced, and get converted. Then you will begin to change. What else needs to happen? Commitment. Being convicted, convinced, converted, and changed does not mean that there will never be a failure. You must be committed to work out this new lifestyle day by day. And if you fail, don't give up, but begin again. You will get stronger each day.

Start by following some of the tips on the next few pages. I hope it will be a practical guide to help you on your journey to a better way of eating.

TIPS FOR HEALTHY EATING

Examine Your Eating Habits
Write down everything you eat for one or two weeks. Soon you'll see a pattern of unhealthy habits you need to break.

Write Down Your Main Nutritional Problem Areas

- Snacking between meals
- Drinking or eating too many caffeinated products (cokes, coffee, chocolate, etc.)
- Eating fried foods
- Eating junk food
- Eating too much meat
- Eating salads with an excess of salad dressing
- Not eating salads
- Eating vegetables drenched with butter or sour cream
- Not eating vegetables
- Other

Subscribe to a Nutrition Magazine or E-mail Newsletter

Examples:

- *American Institute for Cancer Research NEWSLETTER*, 1759 R Street NW, Washington, DC, 20009; AICR Nutrition Hotline:1-800-843-8114; http://www.aicr.org.
- *Bragg NEWS-GRAM: Live Food Products*, Box 7, Santa Barbara, CA, 93102; http://www.bragg.com.
- *HEALTH Magazine*, HEALTH, P. O. Box 56863, Boulder, CO, 80322-6863.
- *Mayo Clinic Health Source*, 200 First Street SW, Rochester, MN, 55905; http://www.mayohealth.org.
- *Nutrition Action Healthletter*, CSPI, 1875 Conn. Ave. NW, Suite 300, Washington, DC, 20009; E-Mail: circ@cspinet.org; http://www.cspinet.org/nah.
- *Prevention Magazine*, P. O. Box 7319, Red Oak, IA, 51591-0319; http://www.healthyideas.com.

Buy a Good Cookbook.

Examples:

- *Cooking for Life*, Gordon S. Tessler
- *Eating for Excellence Cookbook*, Sheri Rose Shepherd
- *No-Stove Nutrition: Recipes and Activities for Healthy Eaters*, Sandy Heffelfinger
- *Set for Life*, Jane P. Merrill and Karen M. Sunderland

- *The 15-Minute Meal Planner: A Realistic Approach to a Healthy Lifestyle*, Sue Gregg and Emilie Barnes
- *The Good Book Cookbook*, Naomi Goodman, Robert Marcus, and Susan Woolhandler
- *The Guilt-Free Comfort Food Cookbook*, Georgia Kostas and Robert Barnett
- *The Rodale Cookbook*, Nancy Albright

Buy a Nutrition Book*
Examples:
- *Advanced Nutritional Therapies*, Dr. Kenneth H. Cooper
- *Does the Bible Teach About Nutrition?*, Elizabeth Baker
- *Eat for the Health of It*, Martha A. Erickson
- *Feel Like a Million*, Dr. Catharyn Elwood
- *Fit Kids*, Dr. Kenneth H. Cooper
- *God's Key to Health and Happiness*, Elmer Josephson
- *Healing Secrets from the Bible*, Patrick Quillan
- *Health and Nutrition*, Kathleen Baldinger
- *Let's Eat Right to Keep Fit*, Adelle Davis
- *Lifelong Health*, Mary Ruth Swope
- *Nutrition Almanac*, John D. Kirschman
- *Prescription for Nutritional Healing*, James F. Balch, M.D. and Phyllis A. Balch, C.N.C.
- *Smart Medicine for Healthier Living*, Janet Zand, L.Ac., Allan N. Spreen, M.D., C.N.C., James B. LaValle, R.Ph., N.D.
- *The Family Nutrition Book*, William Sears, M.D. and Martha Sears, R.N.
- *The World's Oldest Health Plan*, Kathleen O'Bannon Baldinger
- *Vitamin Bible*, Earl Mindell
- *What the Bible Says About Healthy Living*, Rex Russell, M.D.

*These are some of the best resources I have found, but always be discerning and keep a "filter" on your mind. It's difficult to find any book in the nutritional area with which we would totally agree. That is why I have written this book. For in-depth information on any of the subjects covered in this book, please consult a more thorough resource. It is indeed beyond the scope of this work to cover all areas of nutrition exhaustively.

Learn to Shop Wisely in the Grocery Store

- Shop in the sections where good healthy foods are stocked.
- Make a list before you go and stick to it.
- Purchase healthful snacks—fruits, vegetables, decaffeinated fruit drinks, whole grain crackers, etc.
- Read labels (the order of ingredients tells the proportion of that ingredient in relation to other ingredients).
- Cut out or cut down on prepared mixes such as cake mixes and pasta main dishes.
- Cut out or cut down on foods with preservatives (many are cancer-causing).
- Guard your eyes if you must walk through the candy, cookie, or other junk food sections.
- If good and bad foods are stocked together—locate the good products, purchase them, and then immediately go to another aisle.

Shop in a Health Food Store for Some Items

- Whole wheat flour or other whole grain flours
- Wheat berries or other whole grains to grind yourself
- Whole grain pasta (spaghetti, macaroni, lasagna noodles, etc.)
- Cold-pressed cooking oil (olive oil, safflower oil, canola oil, etc.)
- Cold-pressed mayonnaise and salad dressings
- Raw, locally produced honey
- Nuts (raw unsalted almonds, pecans, walnuts, sunflower seeds, soy nuts, pumpkin seeds, cashews, etc.)
- Whole grain crackers and cookies
- Yogurt, plain and frozen
- Sea salt
- Organically grown fruits and vegetables
- Carob powder and carob chips
- Vitamin and mineral supplements
- Sun-dried fruit (raisins, apricots, cranberries, etc.)
- Much, much more

Note: Read labels—even in the health food store. Granted, food in these establishments are likely to be free of harmful additives, but these stores are in business to make money, too. And remember, not every product in the health food store is free of sugar, bad fats, etc. You must watch out for your own health.

Learn the Differences in Fats

- Polyunsaturated—Fatty acids that are usually liquid at room temperature and come from vegetable, nut, or seed sources such as olives, corn, safflowers, and sunflowers.

- Saturated—Fatty acids that are usually hard at room temperature and come from animal sources (except for coconut oil).

- Monounsaturated—Fatty acids that remain liquid at room and body temperature but that solidify in the refrigerator. They are found in olive, peanut, avocado, and other oils.

Learn the Differences in Carbohydrates

- *Principal Carbohydrates* include sugars, starches, and cellulose. These are the primary sources of energy—necessary for the digestion and assimilation of other foods.

  Sugars—Simple sugars, as in honey and fruits, are easily digested. Double sugars, such as table sugar, require more digestion.

  Starches require prolonged enzymatic action in order to be broken down into simple sugars (glucose) for digestion.

  Cellulose is commonly found in the skins of fruits and vegetables, is largely indigestible by humans, contributes very little energy to the diet, and provides the bulk necessary for intestinal action and elimination.

- *Refined Carbohydrates* include foods such as white flour, white sugar, and white polished rice. They lack B vitamins and other nutrients. "Excessive consumption of these foods will perpetuate any vitamin B deficiency a person may have. If the B vitamins are absent, carbohydrate combustion cannot take place, and indigestion, symptoms of heartburn, and nausea can result. Research continues as to whether or not such problems as diabetes, heart disease, high blood pressure, anemia, kidney disease, and cancer can be linked to an overabundance of refined carbohydrates in the diet. However, a total lack of carbohydrates may produce ketosis, loss of energy, depression, and breakdown of essential body protein," states the *Nutrition Almanac*.

- *Complex Carbohydrates* include natural or unrefined sugars and starches with cellulose. They are naturally found in honey, fruits, whole grains, and vegetables.

Eat Breakfast
Eat whole grain cereals with fruit, or try these breakfasts: bran muffins and a banana smoothie, whole wheat pancakes with maple syrup, whole grain toast with peanut butter, mashed banana with a little honey, or an omelet now and then.

Snack on Fresh Fruits and Vegetables
Keep a bowl filled with fresh fruit on your kitchen counter to encourage healthful snacking. Chop up carrots and celery sticks and keep them in a container of water on the top shelf of your refrigerator.

Fix Healthier Desserts
Desserts can be made healthier by substituting honey for sugar, whole wheat flour for white flour, and oil for shortening. Just remember, cookies, pies, and cakes all have large amounts of ingredients lacking in nutrition and are extremely high in calories.

Eat Fruit for Dessert
Fresh watermelon, peaches, strawberries, blueberries, bananas, and so on are delicious topped with some yogurt or milk. Or try a baked apple or a cluster of grapes served with a piece of cheese.

Make Every Meal Special
Even if it's just bean soup, a salad, and bread, make the meal attractive by setting a pretty table with colorful placemats and flowers. Add a sprig of parsley on each bowl.

Eat More Non-Meat Proteins Than Meat Proteins
- *Cheese*—If you are weight conscious, use skim milk cheese such as mozzarella, farmers, or cottage cheese.
- *Eggs*—These are an excellent source of complete protein; vitamins A, B_2, D, and E; iron; and choline.
- *Legumes*—These include lima beans, black-eyed peas, kidney beans, black beans, navy beans, and lentils.

- Soy products—Tofu, veggie burgers, and soy milk are good sources of protein.

Eat Lots of Vegetables—Raw, Lightly Steamed, or Stir-Fried
Drink at Least Eight Glasses of Purified or Distilled Water Every Day

Eat More Fish
Fish are an excellent source of omega-3 fatty acids. It's best to eat them broiled or baked, and make sure you watch out for fish that are harvested from polluted waters!

Prepare Casseroles or Stir-Fry with a Little Meat and Lots of Vegetables
Bake Your Own Whole Grain Bread, Rolls, and Muffins
Make Your Own Vegetables and Fruit Juices
Grind Wheat Berries and Eat More Brown Rice, Oatmeal, and Other Whole Grains

HOW TO BEGIN

Several years ago I made a radical change in my diet—and the diet of my family. Though my family did not avidly receive these changes at first, they have greatly improved their eating habits over the years.

With some exceptions, I stopped using refined foods (white flour, white rice, white sugar, regular table salt, etc.), carbonated and caffeinated drinks, animal and hydrogenated fats, harmful preservatives, pork and shellfish, and fried foods. In their place I started using whole grains, cold-pressed oils, sea salt, local raw honey (sparingly), filtered drinking water, and fresh vegetable and fruit juices. Although I am still an enthusiastic "believer" in these nutritional practices and more, I realize that I should have adopted these changes more gradually.

With a transition to good eating in mind, I therefore encourage three different levels of nutritional changes (see the next few pages). These are simply my suggestions. Whatever changes you make, however slow or fast, will be wonderful.

LEVEL ONE

Cut Out:

- Animal fat
- Pork (ham, pork chops, pork sausage, bacon, etc.)

Cut Down:

- Carbonated and caffeinated drinks
- Fried foods and snacks (chips, french fries, etc.)
- Desserts made with white sugar, white flour, and hydrogenated shortening
- Sugary snacks between meals (candy, cookies, pastries, etc.)
- Amount of meat eaten (no more than three to four ounces once a day)
- Red meat (no more than three times a week—soak in water one-half hour to help remove blood, sprinkle with kosher salt, rinse, and then broil)
- Amount of salad dressing (not more than one tablespoon per salad serving)
- Sugar-laden cereals and pastries
- Margarine
- Salt (Use sea salt instead.)

Add On:

- Six to eight glasses of purified water a day
- Whole wheat or multigrain bread
- Whole grain cereals
- Brown rice
- More nutritious ingredients in your desserts (Substitute whole wheat flour for white flour, honey for white sugar, oil for shortening, etc.)
- Olive oil instead of other oils for stir-fry, salad dressings, etc.
- Canola or safflower oil instead of other oils for baking
- Stir-fry vegetables (with small amount of meat) at least once a week
- Basket of fresh fruit on your kitchen counter for snacks

- A large, raw vegetable salad at least once a day (Use romaine lettuce, red leaf lettuce, spinach, cauliflower, broccoli, green or red peppers, green onions, cucumbers, black olives, tomatoes, avocados, etc.)
- Vegetable soup once a week
- A green, yellow, or red vegetable at least one meal a day

LEVEL TWO

Cut Out:
- Foods with preservatives

Cut Down:
- Seafood scavengers (shrimp, crab, lobster, catfish, etc.)
- Red meat (no more than once a week)
- Amount of meat (cut down on eating single portion sizes and chop into small pieces for casseroles and stir-fry)
- Carbonated sodas
- Caffeinated drinks

Add On:
- Butter (sparingly) instead of margarine
- Pancakes, muffins, and pastries with whole wheat flour
- Fruits or raw vegetables for snacks
- Whole grain cereals
- Whole wheat or multigrain bread
- Oatmeal (optional—sprinkle with fresh fruit, raisins, nuts, or seeds)
- Dried beans at least twice a week (navy beans, black beans, black-eyed peas, lentils, etc.)
- Stir-fried vegetables at least twice a week with brown rice (optional—add a small amount of chopped chicken)
- Plain yogurt (Make it yourself or choose a store brand without thickeners.)
- Fish at least once a week

LEVEL THREE

Cut Out:

- Seafood scavengers (shrimp, crab, lobster, catfish, etc.)
- Meat that contains antibiotics and growth hormones
- Fried foods
- Red meat (except on rare occasions—remember to soak in water one-half hour to help remove blood, sprinkle with kosher salt, rinse, then broil)
- Cereals, snacks, and desserts made with white sugar and white flour (except on rare occasions)
- Carbonated sodas (except on rare occasions)
- Caffeinated drinks (except on rare occasions)

Cut Down:

- Amount of meat (three to four ounces three to four times a week)

Add On:

- Home-ground whole grains (wheat berries, oatmeal, brown rice, etc.)
- Whole grain pancakes, waffles, and bread
- Soy products as an alternative protein, i.e., tofu, veggie burgers, soy nuts, and soy milk
- Three to five fresh fruits every day, plus an apple
- Fresh vegetable salad two times a day—at least five to seven fresh vegetables each day
- Your own "juiced" fresh vegetables and fruits
- A vinegar/honey cocktail every day (one tablespoon of apple cider vinegar with one tablespoon honey in six ounces of water. Paul Bragg's Apple Cider Vinegar from the health food store is good.)
- Homemade yogurt
- Homegrown alfalfa sprouts

SPIRITUAL APPLICATION

Dr. J. Sidlow Baxter was a wonderful Bible teacher and author who has had a great influence on my life spiritually. He was also a follower of good nutrition and a healthful lifestyle in general. He was in his nineties when he died, and he maintained a tremendous quality of life into his old age. The following is a summary statement of his philosophy of the proper way of eating. He practiced biblical principles for many years.

> How important is proper diet! How many thousands today are in our overcrowded hospitals who never would have been there but for wrong eating! How many have inadvertently committed slow suicide with their knives and forks! Many of us have so perverted and enslaved our palates by devitalized taste-tickling dainties and savories, that to eat food just as Nature supplies it now seems abnormal!
>
> With my Bible open before me I would say to all: keep off meat with the blood still in it. Keep off animal fats. Keep off all parts of the hog. Keep off all those forbidden land creatures and finless aquatic creatures which the Mosaic law disallows. Keep away as much as possible from white bread, white sugar, white rice. Look carefully at the wrapped, packaged or canned foodstuffs which you buy at the grocery stores. Keep away from all those sugary breakfast cereals which tell you the vitamins or minerals which the manufacturer has injected, but do not tell you all the vital elements which have been eliminated.
>
> Even if it costs more, get guaranteed whole-wheat bread; and as a cereal get pure wheat germ. Let the milk which you buy be that which is least artificially treated. Guard against buying those eating commodities which are marked as containing chemical preservatives, also those which have artificial flavorings and colourings.[1]

I'm Free from the Law

I realize that there are various opinions concerning the issues I've discussed in this book. Interpretations of Scripture vary among godly people. I only ask you to have an open mind and heart to evaluate what I have presented.

I have chosen to live by the following biblical principle: "Do you have faith? Have it to yourself before God. Happy is he who does not condemn himself in what he approves. But *he who doubts is condemned if he eats,* because he does not eat from faith; for whatever is not from faith is sin" (Romans 14:22-23, italics mine).

Some issues related to healthful eating are doubtful to me. But if I have doubts, I refrain from certain actions until I am convinced they are right, not the other way around. You must decide for yourself. Just remember, we are not under the law but under grace. Praise God!

I'm Free to Choose the Good

I'm free! I don't follow rules and laws to gain favor with God or to win my salvation. I'm free to do that which is right and good! However, just because I am no longer in bondage to the law doesn't mean I'm free to eat things that harm my body. Yes, now I'm free to choose the good. I now have the power available to carry out that choice.

As a Christian, the Holy Spirit of God lives in me. My body is the temple of the Holy Spirit. I want to glorify God in my body and in my spirit—which both belong to God. First Corinthians 6:20 says, "For you were bought at a price; therefore glorify God in your body and in your spirit, which are God's." If I am filled with His Holy Spirit, I will have self-control in my life. Indeed, I will be under His control.

Power for Living

If we are to overcome any area of weakness in our lives, we must tap into God's power. The only way we can resist temptation and make good choices is through and from the Holy Spirit. Philippians 4:13 gives us this promise: "I can do all things *through* Christ who strengthens me" (italics mine). Where does the power come from when you need to push away from the table or turn down sugary, fat-filled delicacies? It is from the Glory above and the Glory within—Jesus! He gives you the power to be self-controlled.

Sometimes I think that self-control isn't really the best way to describe what we do when we fight temptation. Rather, I think it should be called "Spirit-control," since He is the power source for our victory. Self-control is one of the fruits of the Holy Spirit (see Galatians 5:23). It is what blooms when we are abiding and growing in the Vine of Jesus.

So where do you get the power? You must come to Him. You must acknowledge that *He* has the power to resist temptation—*not you.* You must also repent of a wrong appetite and gluttonous eating if you have been sinning in these ways. Ask God to fill your life and give you overcoming power.

Remember, if you are a Christian, God lives in your body. First John 4:15 says, "Whoever confesses that Jesus is the Son of God, God abides *in him*, and he *in God*" (italics mine). You belong to Him. First Corinthians 6:19-20 says, "Or do you not know that your body is the temple of the Holy Spirit who is in you, whom you have from God, and *you are not your own?* For *you were bought at a price;* therefore glorify God in your body and in your spirit, which are God's" (italics mine). You should greatly desire to take care of your body and to glorify Him in everything you eat or drink.

Therefore, whether you eat or drink, or whatever you do, do all to the glory of God. (1 Corinthians 10:31)

APPENDIX ONE

EAT A VARIETY OF FOODS

God has provided a wide spectrum of delicious foods for us to eat. Each one is unique in its flavor, consistency, and food value. We need to eat a variety of foods to maintain a balanced diet. The guidelines provided by the U.S. Department of Agriculture and U.S. Department of Health and Human Services will enable us to eat the right amounts from each of the five major food groups.

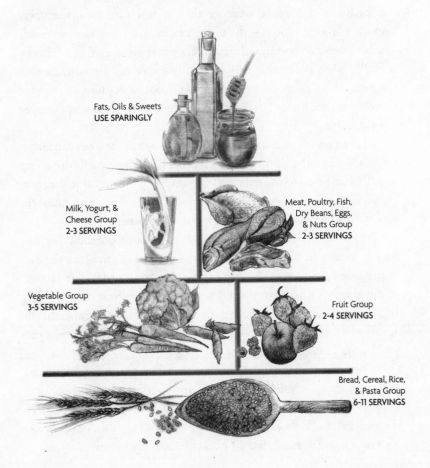

Fats, Oils & Sweets
USE SPARINGLY

Milk, Yogurt, &
Cheese Group
2-3 SERVINGS

Meat, Poultry, Fish,
Dry Beans, Eggs,
& Nuts Group
2-3 SERVINGS

Vegetable Group
3-5 SERVINGS

Fruit Group
2-4 SERVINGS

Bread, Cereal, Rice,
& Pasta Group
6-11 SERVINGS

EATING GOOD—OVEREATING NOT GOOD

There are foods that are bad for you and foods that are good for you. But even too much good food isn't good for you. Remember what they say about too much of a good thing? Well, I think that food is certainly included! The Bible calls that gluttony. Proverbs 23:1-3 says: "When you sit down to eat with a ruler, consider carefully what is before you; and put a knife to your throat if you are a man given to appetite. Do not desire his delicacies, for they are deceptive food."

The phrase "put a knife to your throat" was the way people in biblical times spoke when they urged someone to "curb your appetite" or "control yourself." It is like the phrase we use today: "Bite your tongue." The word *appetite* is also translated "gluttony."

Each of us has a food weakness that tends to offer greater temptation than all other foods—such as sweets because they taste so good. Truth is, they can become addictive. Have you ever heard of a "chocoholic?" Unless we can eat this food only rarely, it's probably best to leave it alone. I rarely eat even "healthful" cookies because it's too easy for me to eat too many. I'm better off leaving sweets alone except on special occasions.

I have a friend who is very health conscious, but she loves chocolate. Once a week, and only once, she eats chocolate. It's probably not going to hurt her because she eats well the rest of the time. But if eating sweets is your daily habit, especially if you're not eating other healthful foods, it will probably cause serious health problems.

It's also easy to eat too much meat. Now you may question that, but let me assure you that most meat portions served at restaurants and in many homes are twice the size of what we truly need. The recommended portion of meat should be about two to four ounces—any bigger and you're eating more than you need! The Bible specifically speaks of "gluttonous eaters of meat" (Proverbs 23:20). Let's make sure we don't fall into that category!

Other foods that can become problematic for us are salty snacks. How easy it is to overindulge in chips, french fries, salted nuts, or popcorn! We do it without thinking! We sit down to watch a movie or sporting event and blindly reach into the bowl or box in front of us. Before we know it, we've finished off a bucket or bowl by ourselves!

The one type of food that is probably impossible for us to overeat is raw vegetables. They're very filling and take longer to chew! Sit down to a raw salad filled with cauliflower, broccoli, tomatoes, carrots, green onions, lettuce, and cucumber, and you're going to have a satisfied feeling after you finish. Here's another good suggestion: Eat a large fresh salad at the beginning of lunch and supper, and you won't eat as much of the other foods.

It's a choice we each must make. Good choices turn into good habits. It's up to you. Choose the "oh, so good."

THE "ALL FOODS ARE CREATED EQUAL" MYTH

There is a nutrition myth being circulated that says: All foods are created equal by God, and nothing is really bad for you. The supporters of this myth say that you can eat whatever you want—just don't eat too much.

I agree to the latter point—we shouldn't overeat. The Bible clearly states in Proverbs 28:7 and 23:20 that we are not to even keep company with gluttons. And in Proverbs 23:2 a glutton is described as someone given to appetite: "And put a knife to your throat if you are a man given to appetite."

But I disagree that you can eat whatever you want—all foods are not created equal. In fact, many foods we eat are not as God originally created—they have been refined by man. The bread that was the staff of life in Bible times was not made with white flour. Indeed, white sugar and hydrogenated shortening are modern discoveries as well. These were made for shelf life, not for our life.

There are many principles for good eating in the Bible, but as in the sciences, God has left many details for man to discover. And we should study those details with a discerning spirit—always remembering that they are not infallible like God's Word. And we should study them with an open mind, knowing that new things are always being discovered—some of which negate what was previously "known."

Ask God to show you the truth about the confusing and seemingly contradictory issues. As you allow God's Word to be your guide, I pray He will make your path straight.

Indulge yourself once a week with one of your favorite desserts. If you're eating well the rest of the time, it won't hurt you. And psychologically this will be a satisfying treat.

Acid-Alkaline Balance

One vital subject in the nutritional field that has been overlooked is the importance of eating foods that have a proper acid-alkaline balance. Many physical ailments are caused by our bodies being too acidic. Instead of eating more alkaline-producing foods, we reach for an antacid to temporarily relieve our discomfort.

To be fair, some acidic foods are good for you when consumed in the proper balance of other food. But some of them are bad for you and should either be eliminated or eaten on a very limited basis. We should learn what foods and drinks are acid-producing and correct this problem. A simplified list of these foods follows.

Acid-Forming	Alkaline-Forming
meat	honey
tea	vegetables:
coffee	tomatoes
carbonated drinks, regular & diet	turnip greens
fats	broccoli
potatoes	green beans
pastries	cauliflower
corn	green, red peppers
dairy products	carrots
flour	onions
pasta	beets
legumes	cabbage
rice	celery
candy	lettuce, all kinds
sugar	mushrooms
green peas	sprouts
green lima beans	fruit:
	apples
	bananas
	oranges
	grapefruit
	watermelon
	cantaloupe
	honeydew melon
	kiwi
	mangoes

Appendix Two

CALORIES AND FAT GRAMS DO COUNT

Some contend that you don't need to count calories or fat grams. They insinuate that keeping track places you in bondage. Yes, you can be in bondage to these things, but being in bondage and being aware are two different things. We should not dismiss the importance of knowing about the calorie and fat composition of our food.

Just as you need a basic knowledge of mathematics to keep your budget balanced, you need a general knowledge of calories and fat grams to make sure your diet is balanced. This knowledge will not place you in bondage to these things. Just the opposite will happen. It will free you. When you have mastered this basic knowledge, your eating and shopping will be on "auto pilot"—you'll be so programmed to this information that you will spend very little time thinking about it.

Where do you start? With the elementary facts. Just as you learned your numbers and multiplication tables, you're going to have to learn basic information about the essentials of fats and calories. Once you've learned the essentials, then you can advance to more in-depth nutritional knowledge.

There is much ignorance on the important subject of nutrition. In addition, a great deal of error and confusion exist in this field; so much of what we have learned isn't true.

As in any area of life—whether it is religion, politics, science, or nutrition—we are personally responsible for discovering and following the truth. I challenge you to search out the truth for yourself. Begin and end with the Bible, though it is not a textbook on nutrition. You won't discover specific details for calorie or fat grams within its pages, but you will be surprised at how much you will discover on the vital subject of healthful eating.

I have listed the calories and fat grams of some common foods. This is strictly an introduction, and I encourage you to purchase a book with a more extensive listing. It will be well worth the investment as you learn the calories and fat grams for the foods you commonly eat.

I hope that you will discover that some foods are higher in their caloric and fat content than others. For instance, meats, carbohydrates, and fats are the highest in calories and fat grams as a rule; vegetables and fruits are the lowest. With this basic knowledge you'll begin to understand how to balance your eating habits. As you take a quick glance at calorie and fat gram values, it will become obvious why over 50 percent of the American people are overweight.

	CALORIES	FAT GRAMS
BREAD		
French toast	55	.6
Pancakes	104	3.2
Whole wheat bread, 1 piece	55	.6
Whole wheat roll, 1	103	1.1
White roll, 1	113	2.1
Waffle, 1 avg.	206	7.3
CANDY		
Chocolate candy bar, 2 oz.	291	32
Chocolate syrup, 1 Tbs.	49	.4
Fudge, 1 piece 1 in. square	180	5.5
Gumdrop, 1 piece	33	.1
Lollipop, 1 med.	102	0
Peanut brittle, 1 piece	110	4.0
CEREAL		
Bran flakes, 1 c.	143	.4
Oatmeal, 1 c. cooked	130	2.4
Raisin bran, 1 c.	184	.8
Shredded wheat, 1 biscuit	99	.6
CONDIMENTS		
Mayonnaise, 1 Tbs.	101	11.2
Mustard, 1 Tbs.	11	.8

	CALORIES	FAT GRAMS
DAIRY		
Butter, 1 Tbs.	100	11.2
Buttermilk, 1 c. (low fat)	90	.2
Cheddar cheese, 1 oz.	68	7.9
Colby cheese, 1 oz.	110	9.0
Cottage cheese, 1 c. (creamed)	235	9.5
Cream cheese, 1 Tbs.	53	5.3
Margarine, 1 Tbs.	100	11.3
Milk, 1 c. (skimmed)	89	.2
Milk, 1 c. (whole)	159	8.8
Sour cream, 1 oz.	57	5.4
Yogurt, 1 c. (plain, part skim)	125	1.2
DESSERT		
Banana bread, 1 slice	134	3.9
Cake		
Angel food, 1 slice	108	0.1
Devil's food, 1 cupcake		
w/choc. icing	184	8.2
White, 1 slice w/icing	188	7.5
Candy		
Fudge, chocolate, 1-in.	180	5.5
Gumdrop	33	0.1
Jelly beans, 1 oz.	102	0.1
Milk chocolate bar	291	18.0

	CALORIES	FAT GRAMS		CALORIES	FAT GRAMS
Chewing gum	9	0	Italian, 1 Tbs.	83	8.8
Chocolate syrup, 1 Tbs.	49	0.4			
			FRUIT		
Cookies			Apple, 1 med.	76	.8
Assorted, 1 med.	38	1.6	Avocado, 1 sm.	90	8.2
Brownie w/nuts, 1 piece	243	16.0	Banana, 1 med.	128	.3
Chocolate chip, 1 med.	46	2.7	Blueberries, 1 c.	87	.7
Oatmeal, w/raisins	90	3.1	Cantaloupe 1/4	30	.1
Vanilla wafer, 1 avg.	23	0.8	Cranberry juice, 1 c.	163	2.5
Gelatin, 1 c. (fruit-flavored)	141	0	Grapefruit, 1 med.	108	.3
Ice cream, 1 c.	389	24.0	Grapes, 1 c.	102	.2
Ice milk, 1 c.	289	9.7	Grape juice, 1 c.	165	trace
Cream puffs, Eclairs, custard	249	14.9	Orange, 1 med.	88	.4
			Orange juice, 1 c.	120	0
Doughnut			Peach, 1 med.	43	.3
Cake	129	5.1	Peaches, 1 c. (in syrup)	201	.3
Raised or yeast	136	8.8	Strawberries, 1 c. (raw)	55	.7
Raised, jelly-filled	226	8.8	Strawberries, 1 c. sliced,		
			sweetened	247	.4
Jams and Jellies, 1 tsp.	54	trace	Watermelon, 4 in. x 8 in.	241	1.8
Pie (1/6 slice from 9-in. pie)					
Apple	346	15.0	**MEAT**		
Boston cream	323	10.0	*Chicken (4 oz.)*		
Cherry	352	15.0	Breast w/skin, fried	230	7.2
Custard	278	14.0	Breast w/skin, baked		
Meringue, chocolate	302	14.0	or broiled	154	4.2
Meringue, lemon	306	12.0	*Fish (4 oz.)*		
Pecan	472	26.0	Cod, broiled	185	6.0
Pumpkin	274	15.0	Salmon, baked or broiled	206	8.2
Strawberry	337	13.0	Snapper, baked or broiled	105	10.2
			Tuna w/oil, drained	213	9.2
Pudding			*Beef (4 oz.)*		
Milk, bread, raisins, 1 c.	468	15.0	Hamburger, lean, broiled	188	9.7
Milk, vanilla, 1 c.	275	9.7	Hamburger, broiled	190	17.2
			Roast, chuck, roasted	370	27
Sherbet, orange, 1 c.	237	2.1	Round steak, broiled	214	6.9
Turnover, 1 avg.	112	4.6	T-bone, broiled	462	39
Whipped topping, 1 Tbs.	13	9.0			
			Lamb (4 oz.) w/fat removed	316	21.2
FAT					
Butter, 1 Tbs.	100	11.2	**NUTS**		
Margarine, 1 Tbs.	100	11.3	Peanuts, 1 c.	1,397	107.0
Oil of any kind, 1 Tbs.	124	14.0	Pecans, 1 c.	715	74.0
Salad Dressing			Pumpkin seeds, 1 c.	1,271	107.0
Blue cheese, 1 Tbs.	76	7.7			

	CALORIES	FAT GRAMS		CALORIES	FAT GRAMS
Sunflower seeds, 1 c.	560	43.0	Beets, 1 c.	39	.4
Walnuts, 1 c.	560	43.0	Broccoli, 1 c.	39	.4
			Cabbage, 1 c.	34	.3
PASTA			Carrots, 1 lge. raw	42	0
Macaroni and cheese, 1 c.	468	24.0	Carrots, 1 c. (cooked)	47	.3
Spaghetti w/meat sauce, 1 c.	335	12.0	Cauliflower, 1 c.	27	.2
			Green beans, 1 c.	31	.2
SOFT DRINKS			Green peas, 1 c.	66	.3
Cola drinks, 12 oz.	140	0	Green pepper, 1 lge.	22	.2
			Lettuce, 3 1/2 oz.	18	.3
SWEETENERS			*Potato*		
Honey, 1 Tbs.	64	0	Baked, 1 med.	93	.1
Molasses, 1 Tbs.	20	0	French fries, 1 c.	329	15.8
Syrup, 1 Tbs.	20	0	Mashed, 1 c.		
Sugar			w/butter, milk	188	8.6
1 Tbs.	46	0	Sweet, 1 med.	141	.5
1 c.	770	0			
VEGETABLES					
Asparagus, 4 spears	12	trace			

The above was gleaned from the *Nutrition Almanac,* which also provides information about the vitamins, minerals, protein, etc., in a large variety of foods. The book can be purchased at your local health food store.

Recipes

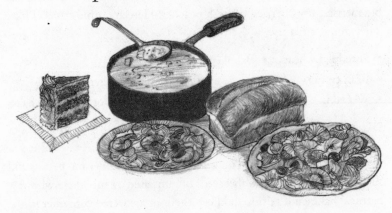

good . . . and good for you

CEREALS AND BREADS

As I mentioned in chapter 2, bread is the "staff of life." But not white bread! I'm referring to bread made with delicious whole grains. I try to make my own bread and grind the wheat berries and other grains. But life gets "oh, so busy" sometimes. When I don't have time, I buy whole grain bread from a local bakery or health food store (both bake the best quality and most delicious bread). I know it costs more than what I would pay at a grocery store, but there is no comparison to the health benefits and delicious taste!

I've included my favorite whole grain bread and pancake recipes (Adrian loves the pancakes). In my humble opinion, you must use buttermilk to make pancakes—there's just no denying what it does to make a fluffier, richer-tasting pancake. I've also included a couple of "quick bread" recipes you might enjoy, as well as my favorite corn bread recipe (also referred to as spoon bread).

CEREALS

Buy only whole grain cereals without added sugar. Top with bananas, blueberries, strawberries, or fresh peaches! Here are some cereals I like. They are worth a try.

- Shredded wheat
- Bran cereal
- Weetabix
- Whole grain Cheerios
- Uncle Sam's cereal with flax seed
- Whole grain oat, corn, wheat, or multigrain flakes

Nuts, Seeds, Oatmeal, Raisin Mix

I buy the following items in bulk—nuts such as walnuts and pecans and sunflower, pumpkin, and flax seeds (all unsalted). I mix these with raw oatmeal flakes and raisins and keep them in a covered container in the freezer. When I serve cereal, I pour some into a small bowl to thaw. Then I serve it as an accompaniment. Just remember—though this mixture is loaded with good things such as omega-3 oils, it's also packed with calories—so don't eat too much on your cereal! This mixture is also handy as an added bonus in your pancake, waffle, and bread batter or sprinkled over some yogurt.

Oatmeal

I serve hot oatmeal several times a week. It helps lower cholesterol. Cook as directed on the box and top with local raw honey, a spoonful of mixed nuts, seeds, or raisins. Add sliced bananas, blueberries, or other fresh fruit. You can serve it with or without milk. You may even want to try soy milk for a change. It's full of those good isoflavones.

BREADS

Whole Grain Bread

5 c.	hot tap water	3 Tbs.	Rapid Rise yeast
⅔ c.	honey	⅔ c.	oil
1½	Tbs. salt	11-14 c.	whole grain flour*
¼ c.	gluten flour or 2 Tbs. dough enhancer		

Combine water and yeast in container for about ten minutes and let yeast dissolve until bubbly. Combine this mixture with oil, honey, and salt in a mixing bowl. Using the lowest mixer speed, slowly add flour until the dough leaves the sides and bottom of bowl. Secure lid, turn to a higher speed. Knead for six minutes. Let dough rise for thirty minutes. Punch it down and shape into loaves and place into greased bread pans. Put in 150°F oven until double in bulk (about thirty minutes). Increase oven to 350°F and bake from thirty-five to forty minutes or until brown. Remove from pans and cool on rack.

*May substitute 1 c. rice flour, 1 c. barley flour, 1 c. soy flour, 1 c. oat flour or oatmeal.

Whole Wheat Pancakes

2	eggs
2 tsp.	baking powder
1 tsp.	baking soda
1 tsp.	salt
2 c.	whole wheat flour (substitute ½ c. oatmeal flour for extra lightness)
2¼ c.	buttermilk (adjust amount of buttermilk for thickness or thinness of pancakes)
2 Tbs.	oil (substitute 2 heaping Tbs. of applesauce for no-fat)

Beat eggs and stir in dry ingredients and oil. Use butter sparingly and top with pure maple syrup or a spoonful of plain yogurt with orange marmalade or blueberries, bananas, or strawberries for a gourmet delight. (Or sometimes indulge in a topping of real whipped cream with sprinkled nuts.)

Zucchini Bread

2 c.	all-purpose flour (or 1:1 white/whole wheat)		1 c.	canola or safflower oil
			3	large eggs
1 tsp.	salt		2 c.	sugar or 1½ c. honey
2 tsp.	cinnamon		1 Tbs.	vanilla extract
¼ tsp.	ground cloves		1 c.	walnuts, finely chopped
½ tsp.	allspice		2 c.	zucchini, grated
2 tsp.	baking soda			
1 tsp.	baking powder			

Optional:
½ c.   grated coconut

Preheat oven to 350°F. Butter and flour two eight-inch loaf pans. Sift flour, cinnamon, ground cloves, allspice, baking soda, baking powder, and salt together in a bowl. In a separate bowl, beat eggs until frothy. Add sugar, oil, and vanilla to eggs and continue beating until smooth and thick. Alternate adding one-third of dry ingredients and one-third of grated zucchini; mix between each addition. Repeat until both are incorporated. Fold in chopped walnuts. Put dough into loaf pans and bake about one hour or until a toothpick comes out clean.

Yogurt Cornbread

1 can	creamed corn (8.5 oz.)		½ c.	canola oil
1 c.	plain yogurt		1 c.	self-rising cornmeal
2	eggs		2 tsp.	baking powder

Preheat oven to 400°F. Add a little oil to an iron skillet and put skillet in oven. Combine corn, yogurt, eggs, and oil; beat well. Combine cornmeal and baking powder and add to corn mixture. Pour into hot iron skillet. Bake for thirty minutes or until well done. Test by putting a sharp knife into the middle. If the knife comes out clean, the cornbread is ready.

Spoon Bread

1½ c.	boiling water		1 c.	white cornmeal
1 tsp.	salt		1 tsp.	baking powder
¼ tsp.	baking soda		1 Tbs.	butter, softened
3	eggs, separated		1 c.	buttermilk
1 tsp.	honey			

Preheat oven to 375°F. Grease a two-quart casserole dish. Beat egg whites until soft peaks form; set aside. In a large bowl, stir boiling water into cornmeal. To prevent lumping, continue stirring mixture until it is cool. Blend in butter and egg yolks. Stir in buttermilk, salt, honey, baking powder, and baking soda. Fold beaten egg whites into batter. Pour into casserole dish. Bake forty-five to fifty minutes. Insert knife in center to see if it's done. Serve hot. Ummm good!

Carrot-Raisin Bread

3 c.	flour*		1	small can crushed pineapple
2 tsp.	baking soda		2 c.	grated carrots
1 tsp.	salt		1 c.	chopped pecans or walnuts
3 tsp.	cinnamon		½ c.	raisins
1½ c.	canola or safflower oil		2 tsp.	pure vanilla extract
1¼ c.	honey		3	eggs

Drain the pineapple. Mix together all ingredients and pour into two greased loaf pans. Bake at 325° F for about one hour.

*Or 1 c. unbleached white and 2 c. whole wheat flour.

DESSERTS

Desserts made from sugar and other rich ingredients should not be a part of our daily diets. Instead delicious fresh fruit can be a tasty end to a healthful meal.

When my husband and I were in Taiwan on a mission trip, we were served wonderful pineapples, mangoes, melons, bananas, and other fresh fruit at every meal. The closest thing to what we might call a dessert was a sweet potato casserole. Now why do I mention this? Because Asians, with their diet of fresh fruit, stir-fried vegetables, and small amounts of meat have a much lower cancer rate than those of us in the West. Studies have shown that when Asians move to the West and adopt our eating habits, their cancer rate increases.

It's going to take a lot for Westerners to choose a healthier way to end a meal, because our palates have grown accustomed to sugar-laden dainties. But I don't think it's impossible to retrain our taste buds. Let me add that indulging in one of the "delicious dainties" from time to time won't hurt you if you eat healthful food most of the time. One of these indulgences is Mama's Sour Cream Cake. Although she has gone to heaven, I still have her recipe that she gave me in her own handwriting.

For over twenty years, I have tried to prepare more nutritious desserts for friends and family. I have included some of these here.

Baked Custard

3 eggs	slightly beaten	⅓ c.	mild honey
	dash of salt	2½ c.	milk, scalded
1 tsp.	pure vanilla extract		nutmeg

Preheat oven to 350°F. Blend eggs, honey, salt, and vanilla. Gradually stir in milk. Pour into six six-ounce custard dishes or one large dish. Sprinkle with nutmeg. Place dishes in a larger baking pan. Create a hot water bath for custard dish(es) by pouring hot water into the larger pan within ½ inch of the tops of the custard dish(es). Bake about forty-five minutes or until a knife inserted halfway between the center and the edge comes out clean. Remove dishes from water and serve custard warm or chilled. Sprinkle with nutmeg.

Honey Oatmeal Cookies

¾ c.	canola or safflower oil	1¼ c.	honey
2 tsp.	pure vanilla extract	2	eggs
¾ c.	powdered milk	½ c.	raisins
½ c.	chopped walnuts	1½ c.	wheat germ
¾ c.	whole wheat flour	1 tsp.	salt
1 c.	unsweetened coconut, fine-grated	2 c.	rolled oats

Preheat oven to 350°F. In a large mixing bowl, combine the oil, honey, eggs, and vanilla. Beat till thoroughly mixed. Stir in the coconut, raisins, chopped nuts, wheat germ, and rolled oats—stirring until evenly blended. In a separate bowl, stir together the whole wheat flour with the dry powdered milk and salt. Add to the cookie dough and stir until the mixture is smooth. Push from a teaspoon onto a greased cookie sheet. Bake for ten to twelve minutes. Remove hot cookies from the cookie sheet immediately and cool on paper towels. Yield: about four dozen cookies.

Fruity Yogurt Parfaits

large container of nonfat plain Yogurt		honey to taste
fresh fruit, chopped	2 c.	granola

Stir honey into yogurt to give it a "sweet to taste" flavor. Spoon yogurt/honey mixture into parfait glasses. Layer fruit and granola on alternative layers. For Fourth of July, this is especially pretty with blueberries and strawberries.

Scripture Cake

2 c.	all purpose flour (or 1 c. whole wheat pastry flour)		
½ c.	butter	¾ c.	molasses
½ tsp.	baking soda	½ tsp.	ground cinnamon
¼ tsp.	ground cloves	⅛ tsp.	ground ginger
3 eggs	beaten	½ c.	buttermilk
⅓ c.	honey	½ to 1 c.	raisins
1 c.	dried figs, chopped	½ c.	almonds, chopped
½ c.	orange juice		

Preheat oven to 325°F. In large mixing bowl cream butter until light; blend in molasses. Stir together flour, baking soda, cinnamon, cloves, ginger, and a dash of salt. Combine eggs, buttermilk, and honey. Add egg mixture and dry ingredients alternately to creamed mixture. Stir in raisins, figs, and almonds. Turn mixture into greased and floured 9x5x3 loaf pan. Bake for forty minutes. Loosely cover with foil. Bake fifty minutes more. Let cool in pan ten minutes; remove from pan. Cool on rack; brush all sides with orange juice. Wrap in foil and store twelve days in refrigerator. Makes one loaf.

Jewish Apple Cake

(Baked by Lynn Sherwood)

3 c.	flour (2 c. white, 1 c. whole wheat)		
1½ c.	honey	¼ c.	orange juice
1 c.	canola or safflower oil	2½ tsp.	vanilla extract
4	eggs	3 tsp.	baking powder
½ tsp.	salt	1 c.	nuts, chopped

Filling:

2 c.	thinly sliced apples	2 tsp.	sugar
1 tsp.	cinnamon		

Preheat oven to 350°F. Beat the eggs, sugar, oil, juice, and vanilla at high speed for ten minutes. Blend in dry ingredients, which have been sifted together, a little at a time. Fold in nuts. Put one-third of the batter into a well-greased bundt pan. Arrange half of the filling on the batter. Cover with second third of the batter. Alternate the second half of the filling and top with the last third of the batter. Bake for one hour and fifteen minutes. Sprinkle with powdered sugar while still warm.

Prune Bars

¾ c.	whole wheat pastry flour	1 c.	diced prunes
1 c.	chopped walnuts	1½ tsp.	baking powder
1 c.	firmly packed date sugar	¼ tsp.	salt
3	eggs, slightly beaten		

Preheat oven to 325°F. Combine prunes, walnuts, date sugar, flour, baking powder, and salt; mix thoroughly. Add eggs, blending well. Spread dough evenly in a greased nine-inch-square pan. Bake about thirty minutes or until done. Cut into bars and roll in powdered sugar.

Pumpkin Bars

⅔ c.	butter	2 tsp.	cinnamon
2 c.	honey	½ tsp.	ginger
3	eggs	½ tsp.	cloves
1 can	pumpkin, 16 oz.	2 tsp.	baking powder
2 c.	whole wheat flour	½ tsp.	salt
½ tsp.	baking soda		

Icing:

8 oz. cream cheese, softened and sweetened with honey to taste

Preheat oven to 325°F. Cream butter and honey; blend in eggs and pumpkin. Combine dry ingredients and add to wet mixture; stir thoroughly. Pour mixture into greased 15½ x 10½ x ½ jelly roll pan or cookie sheet. Bake for thirty-five to forty minutes or until a toothpick inserted in the center comes out clean. Cool. Beat cream cheese and honey and frost the bars. Garnish with pecan halves, if desired. Chopped nuts may be added to the pumpkin bar mixture before baking.

Banana Oatmeal Krispies

2 c.	oatmeal		¼ c.	honey
½ c.	canola or safflower oil		½ c.	coconut flakes
½ c.	raisins		¾ c.	dates, chopped
1 tsp.	salt		1 tsp.	vanilla extract
1	ripe banana, mashed			

Preheat oven to 350°F. Mix honey and oil with oatmeal. Let stand. Mix remaining ingredients and combine with honey mixture. Drop by teaspoons onto cookie sheet and bake for fifteen to twenty minutes.

FAVORITE CAKES FOR SPECIAL OCCASIONS

(Not entirely healthy, but oh, so good!)

Mama's Sour Cream Cake

2	sticks butter, softened		3 c.	sugar
6	medium eggs (or 4 large)		1 c.	sour cream
3 c.	flour		½ tsp.	baking soda
1 tsp.	baking powder		¼ tsp.	salt

Preheat oven to 350°F. Beat butter and sugar. Add eggs one at a time, beating between each addition. Into a separate bowl, sift flour with soda, salt, and baking powder. Alternate between adding flour mixture and sour cream to the batter until completely blended. Bake for fifty minutes. Take out of oven and turn onto a cooling rack immediately.

Carrot Cake

2 c.	flour		2 c.	sugar
2 tsp.	baking powder		1½ c.	canola oil
2 tsp.	baking soda		4	eggs
2 tsp.	cinnamon, heaping		3 c.	carrots, grated
¾ c.	pecans or walnuts, chopped		1 tsp.	salt

Preheat oven to 300°F. In a large mixing bowl, beat oil, sugar, and eggs until light and fluffy. Add grated carrots gradually and stir. Sift flour with baking powder, baking soda, salt, and cinnamon into a smaller bowl and then stir in chopped nuts. Stir dry ingredients into wet ingredients by hand until well blended. Pour into a lightly greased and floured 9x13 loaf pan or two nine-inch cake pans. Bake for thirty to thirty-five minutes. Use a toothpick to test for doneness. Cool for about ten minutes on a cake rack.

Icing:

4 Tbs.	butter (½ stick), melted		8 oz.	cream cheese*
2 tsp.	pure vanilla extract		2 c.	powdered sugar

Beat all ingredients until fluffy. Spread on cooled cake. For best results, use cream cheese directly from the refrigerator instead of at room temperature. Use two recipes for one three-layer cake. Store cake in refrigerator to preserve moistness.

*Fat-free cream cheese doesn't work.

DRINKS

As you have figured out by now, pure water is my drink of choice. From time to time I also enjoy juicing my own fresh vegetables and fruits. There are endless combinations, but the best I've discovered is carrots with either celery, beets, or apples. Of course, I recommend that you don't substitute drinking juices for water.

Also you might want to try fruit smoothies prepared with milk, yogurt, or buttermilk (my husband loves the buttermilk/fruit combination). Plain buttermilk is not something I favor drinking by itself, but I really like it for a fruit smoothie. Another suggestion is one my husband enjoys—adding "sparkling water" to his favorite fruit juice. You might like it, too!

Finally, there is a lot to be said about the value of drinking tea— especially ginseng or other herbal teas. You might want to check these out next time you're perusing the coffee/tea grocery store aisle. Some herbal teas are a source of healthful antioxidants. Here are a few other refreshing drink ideas:

Fruit Smoothie

½ c.	plain yogurt (or milk)	2-3	ice cubes
½ c.	diced fresh fruit, such as a banana, peach, or strawberries		

Place all ingredients in a blender and puree until smooth. You can substitute frozen fruit for the ice cubes.

Fruit Tea

(As served by Vicki Mullins)

1 qt.	water	6 oz.	frozen lemonade concentrate
1	family-size tea bag	6 oz.	frozen limeade concentrate
½ c.	mild honey	½ can	pineapple juice

Microwave tea bags in water for six minutes. Let steep for ten minutes. Add concentrates, juice, and honey. Add an additional quart of water and enjoy

Slush Punch

12 oz.	frozen orange juice concentrate		juice of 3 lemons
1 c.	pineapple juice	10 c.	cold water
⅔ c.	honey	2	bananas
1 c.	frozen strawberries (partially thawed)		

Mix the punch in a gallon jar. Stir the frozen orange juice together with the pineapple juice and the freshly squeezed lemon juice and the cold water—stirring until mixed. Pour one cup of this juice into your blender along with the honey and two sliced bananas. Process until the bananas are smoothly pureed. Add the bananas to the fruit punch.

Now pour one more cupful of juice in the blender, but this time add the partially thawed strawberries. Process until the strawberries are smoothly pureed and stir them into the fruit punch. Freeze for at least twenty-four hours in an airtight moisture-proof container(s). Remove from the freezer several hours before serving. It should be semi-frozen and thick to be good. Add carbonated beverage just before serving, if desired. Stir and serve in "slush" stage. Ideal for the holidays or any festive occasion. Yield: one gallon

Hot Cranberry Cider

(As served by Faith Anderson)

½ gallon	cranberry juice	1 quart	apple juice
2 sticks	cinnamon		

Combine ingredients in a large saucepan and heat thoroughly. Serve in punch cups.

MEATS

I wrote at length about the subject of meat in the seventh chapter of this book, so I won't reiterate much at this point. Briefly, let me say that God gave us conditions by which He permitted meat to be eaten and enjoyed. He also warned us about being gluttonous eaters of meat. We need to practice moderation and give great effort to preparation. We need to safeguard the preparation of the meat we eat, since modern processing and grazing methods have created some health hazards. And finally eating the right kind of fish is also important. We learned earlier that "fatty" fish, such as salmon, are rich in omega-3 oils. Here are a few of my favorite meat recipes.

Old Fashioned Lamb or Beef Stew

2 lbs.	lamb/beef stew meat	½ c.	whole wheat flour
1 Tbs.	salt	¼ tsp.	pepper
2 Tbs.	olive oil	6 c.	hot water
4	carrots, in 1-in. slices	3	med. potatoes w/skins
1	green pepper, sliced in strips	2-3	med. onions, chopped
2	beef bouillon cubes (optional)	1	bay leaf

Trim fat off stew meat and cut into one-inch cubes. Cut potatoes into one-inch cubes. Mix flour, salt, and pepper. Coat meat with mixture. Heat olive oil in a large skillet and brown meat thoroughly (this can be done faster in a pressure cooker.) Add water and heat to boiling. Reduce heat; cover and simmer two hours. Stir in remaining ingredients. Simmer thirty minutes or until vegetables are tender. If desired, thicken stew (mix 1 cup cold water and two to four tablespoons of flour in jar. Cover, shake, and stir into stew, heat to boiling, stirring constantly. Boil and stir one minute.) Makes six servings.

Variation: Substitute three to four pounds of stewing chicken and chicken bouillon cubes. Cook for two hours or prepare in pressure cooker according to directions.

Cornish Hens

1	Cornish hen (about 1 lb.)	2 Tbs.	orange juice
1½ Tbs.	honey	1½ Tbs.	soy sauce
½ tsp.	ground ginger	2	cloves garlic, crushed
1 Tbs.	apple cider vinegar	1 tsp.	grated orange rind

Preheat oven to 400°F. Prepare marinade by mixing orange juice, honey, soy sauce, ginger, garlic, vinegar, and orange rind in a medium-sized bowl. Brush hen with marinade on inside and outside. Place in a pan and bake for about fifteen minutes. Reduce heat to 350°F and bake an additional thirty to forty-five minutes. Brush with mixture again after thirty minutes. The bird should be golden brown when ready to serve.

Chicken Florentine

(Specialty of Sherrie Angel)

1 10-oz. pkg. frozen chopped spinach (thawed, drained, squeezed dry)

2 c.	cooked chicken	1 can	artichoke hearts, 15 oz.
1 can	cream of chicken soup	½ c.	dry bread crumbs
½ c.	mayonnaise	1 Tbs.	lemon juice
1 tsp.	curry powder	1½ Tbs.	butter, melted
¼ c.	sharp cheddar cheese, shredded		

Preheat oven to 350°F. Spray 9x12 pan with oil. Cut the chicken into pieces. Quarter the artichoke hearts. Layer artichokes, spinach, and chicken in the pan. Combine soup, mayonnaise, lemon juice, and curry powder. Spread over layered mixture. Sprinkle with cheese. Mix bread crumbs and butter and place on top. Bake uncovered thirty minutes.

Honey-Roasted Chicken

2 lbs.	chicken pieces, skinned	1 c.	honey
½ c.	reduced-sodium teriyaki sauce	¼ c.	orange juice
1 Tbs.	Dijon mustard		

Preheat oven to 375°F. Rinse chicken and pat dry. Place in a single layer in a shallow baking dish. In a medium bowl, stir together remaining ingredients. Pour over chicken pieces. Bake uncovered about forty-five minutes or until chicken is tender—basting with honey mixture occasionally.

Chutney Chicken Salad

(My favorite chicken salad)

2	fresh pineapples	2½ c.	cubed chicken breasts
¾ c.	diced celery	1 can	mandarin oranges, 11 oz.
¾ c.	mayonnaise*	2 Tbs.	chutney
1 tsp.	curry	1	medium banana
½ c.	flaked coconut		

Cut pineapples in half. Scoop centers out and cut them into bite-size pieces. Mix pineapple, chicken, celery, mandarin oranges, and mayonnaise (can do this on previous day). Add chutney, curry, banana, and coconut the day of serving, or salad will get grainy and mushy. It does not keep well after mixing in these last ingredients. Serve salad in the pineapple shells.

*Can use light mayo or use half mayo and half plain yogurt.

Recipe from the Women's Ministry, Community Church, Tempe, Arizona.

Salmon

(As offered by my good friend Pat Mason)

1 c.	diced Roma tomatoes	¼ c.	fresh basil
¼ c.	fresh parsley	4 tsp.	capers, rinsed
2-3	crushed garlic cloves	1-2 Tbs.	warm olive oil
lemon	juice to taste	4 pieces	salmon

Marinate salmon in olive oil, salt, pepper, and crushed garlic. Broil or grill four to five minutes per side, or microwave for four to five minutes or until it reaches the desired doneness. Top with tomatoes, basil, parsley, and capers.

Lamb Roast

One of our family's favorite meat dishes is lamb. Preheat oven to 375°F. Prepare meat first by making sure it is free of blood. Next rub the meat with crushed garlic. Then sprinkle with basil and oregano. Salt and pepper to taste. Bake for twenty minutes per pound.

Stuffed Green Peppers

6 lge.	green peppers	5 c.	boiling salted water
1 lb.	ground turkey or soy "ground round"	1 sm.	onion, chopped
1 tsp.	sea salt	1-2	cloves garlic, crushed
1 c.	cooked brown rice	1 can	tomato sauce, 15 oz.

Preheat oven to 350°F. Cut thin slices from stem end of each pepper, remove all seeds and membranes, and wash inside and outside. Cook peppers in the boiling salted water five minutes and then drain (or place green peppers in glass pie dish with about one-fourth inch of water in bottom and microwave for three to five minutes). Cook and stir ground turkey or soy "ground round" and onion in skillet until onion is tender. Drain off any fat. Stir in salt, garlic, rice, and one cup of the tomato sauce; heat through. Lightly stuff each pepper with meat and rice mixture. Stand each upright in ungreased baking dish. Pour remaining tomato sauce over peppers. Cover; bake forty-five minutes. Uncover; bake fifteen minutes longer. Makes six servings.

Strawberry Salsa

(Tangy sauce for chicken or fish)

1 pint	strawberries	3	med. sweet red peppers
2	green med. bell peppers	2	med. tomatoes
1	large Anaheim pepper	¼ c.	chopped cilantro
½ c.	honey	½ c.	fresh lemon juice
½ tsp.	black pepper	1 tsp.	salt
1 tsp.	crushed, dried red chili pepper		

Dice, slice, and remove the seeds from all the fruits and vegetables. Mix together. Refrigerate overnight to allow flavors to blend. Serve over grilled chicken or fish. Makes about one and a half quarts.

OMELETS

I know that eggs have received a "bad rap" for being high in cholesterol. But if you don't overeat them, fresh farm eggs are still nutritious. An omelet filled with cheese and chopped vegetables can make a quick and delicious supper. You can even add chicken or turkey for extra protein. Serve with a salad, fresh fruit, and some good whole wheat toast on the side, and you've got a winning meal!

Spanish (Potato) Omelet

3 med.	potatoes, cubed	1	med. onion, finely chopped
1	clove garlic, crushed	2 Tbs.	fresh parsley, chopped
5	eggs, lightly beaten	3 Tbs.	milk
2 Tbs.	olive oil	1 Tbs.	butter

Optional:

1	lge. red (Spanish) onion, sliced
2	med. banana peppers
	(remove seeds and slice) or a red pepper sliced in "circles"

Cook potatoes in either a pan of boiling water with salt, until just tender, or in a pressure cooker (follow directions). Drain potatoes. Heat butter and oil in a deep nonstick frying pan over medium heat. Add onions, banana peppers, and garlic, and cook five to six minutes or until tender, stirring occasionally. Add potatoes and cook for another five minutes. Remove potatoes and onions to a large bowl. Add chopped parsley and beaten eggs and milk to the potato, pepper, and onion. Mix until well combined. Arrange the red pepper slices over the bottom of a hot, oiled frying pan. Pour the mixture over the peppers, reduce the heat to low and cook, covered, for ten minutes or until the underside is golden. Brown the top of the omelet under a hot grill, if desired.

Note: This omelet is "oh-so-good" served with red leaf lettuce and slices of red onions with black olives and garnished with sprigs of fresh herbs.

Oven Omelet

(As baked by Faith Anderson)

8	eggs	1 c.	milk
8	slices of cheese (any variety)		

Preheat oven to 425°F. Arrange cheese in a greased ten-inch pie tin or shallow casserole dish. Beat eggs with milk. Pour into pan and bake twenty-five to thirty minutes. You can cut down on this proportionately, i.e., six eggs with three-fourths cup milk and six slices of cheese.

A Quick Supper—Veggie/Cheese Omelet

4	eggs, beaten	⅛ c.	milk (low-fat or skim)
½ c.	cheese, grated	½	sm. onion, chopped
¼ tsp.	basil	½ c.	mushrooms, sliced
	salt and pepper to taste		

Optional:

4	asparagus spears	½ c.	broccoli flowerets
1	med. tomato, chopped	1-2	garlic cloves, crushed
4	green onions, chopped		

Beat eggs with milk and pour into skillet—lifting sides of omelet to let uncooked mixture roll under to cook. When done, sprinkle with cheese and fold omelet over to melt cheese. Cover with vegetables and serve.

RICE AND PASTA

Rice and pasta dishes can be served alone or mixed with a multitude of ingredients to be a main course. I eat only brown rice and whole grain pasta at home, but I will eat white rice and other pasta when I go out to eat. I limit my intake of white rice and pasta made with white flour because they have very little food value.

Most grocery stores and all health food stores stock brown rice and whole wheat pasta. One such pasta I have recently been enjoying is orzo. It is a delicious whole grain pasta that requires less cooking time than traditional pasta and rice. I've eaten orzo combined with spinach and herbs in restaurants. What a treat!

Brown rice is especially nutritious. It is rich in the B vitamins, which are so essential for energy. It takes longer to cook (approximately forty-five minutes), so I usually triple the amount I need for my meal and freeze the rest in bags. This way, I can "whip up" a quick meal at a moment's notice. There is an almost endless variety of rice and pasta dishes. Here are a few of my favorites.

Corn, Jalapeño Pepper, Rice Casserole

(As served by Pat Brand)

1 c.	brown rice	1	med. onion, chopped
1	med. green pepper, chopped	1 c.	celery, chopped
1-2	lge. jalapeño peppers, chopped	¼ c.	butter
2 cans	cream-style corn, 17 oz.	1 c.	mild cheddar cheese, grated

Preheat oven to 350°F. Cook rice. Saute vegetables in butter. Add vegetables, rice, cheese, and corn to casserole dish. Cook for forty to forty-five minutes.

Spanish Rice

(As given by Margo Dixon)

1 c.	uncooked brown rice		2 c.	onions, minced
1	green pepper, chopped		1	clove garlic, crushed
½ c.	celery, chopped		¼ c.	olive oil
3 c.	canned tomatoes		1 tsp.	salt
dash	cayenne pepper		¼ lb.	cheddar cheese, grated

Preheat oven to 350°F. Cook rice (according to directions on package). Saute onions, celery, green pepper, and garlic in olive oil. Add tomatoes with juice and salt and pepper. Cook five to six minutes. Combine rice and tomato mixture in three-quart dish. Add cheese to top of casserole. Bake for thirty minutes.

Vegetable Spaghetti

2 Tbs.	olive oil		1	green pepper, chopped
1	lge. onion, chopped		6-8	fresh mushrooms, sliced
1	carrot, grated		1 c.	eggplant, chopped
2	cloves garlic, crushed		1 Tbs.	dried parsley
1 tsp.	basil		½ tsp.	oregano
½ tsp.	thyme		1 jar	tomato pasta sauce, 16 oz.
	salt and pepper to taste			

Optional:
Soy ground round or turkey hamburger

Saute vegetables in oil and spices. Add tomato sauce. Serve over wilted spinach or whole wheat angel hair pasta.

Vegetable Pasta Salad

4 c.	cooked multicolored pasta (tomato, spinach, whole wheat)		
2	carrots, thinly sliced	1	green pepper, chopped
1	lge. Spanish onion, chopped	1	red pepper, chopped
10	fresh mushrooms, sliced	1 tsp.	basil
1	yellow squash, thinly sliced	2	tomatoes, chopped
1 Tbs.	parsley or cilantro		salt and pepper to taste
1	zucchini squash, thinly sliced		

Optional:
Can of tuna fish

Mix all ingredients together (except tomatoes) and chill. Can keep in refrigerator for three to four days. Right before serving add chopped tomatoes.

SALADS

Vegetable Salads

Salads should have a dominant place in our daily diets. But the old stand-by salad of Boston lettuce with chopped tomatoes, cheese, and croutons should be our last resort. That's because Boston lettuce is the least nutritious of all the lettuces. Dark green ones like romaine, red leaf, and green leaf are the best.

I like to keep a supply of these lettuces and spinach in my refrigerator at all times, along with a variety of my favorite raw veggies such as broccoli, cauliflower, green pepper, asparagus, zucchini, and squash. I chop, mix, and sprinkle with a few raw nuts and seeds, and, voila!, I've got the beginnings of a great salad! Now to top it off!

Beware of the trap that many people fall into when they eat salads—too much salad dressing! Don't drench your fresh garden salad with gobs of fattening salad dressing. Remember, one tablespoon of regular dressing can be 100 calories or more. A ladle full of dressing can easily be 500 calories!

On the flip side, I recommend that you get about a tablespoon of good oil in your diet every day. Instead of a mayonnaise and oil-based dressing, I recommend a dressing that has one part oil (olive, canola, soy, etc.) and one part vinegar. If you must have the mayonnaise-based dressing, I suggest that you dilute it with water or vinegar. Mix dressing in a side dish and lightly dip each bite into the saucer before eating. You'll be surprised at how far your dressing will go when it is on the side rather than poured over your salad carte blanche.

Mixed Vegetable Salad

	romaine lettuce		red leaf lettuce
	spinach	1	tomato
½	cucumber	½	green pepper
½ c.	broccoli flowerets	½ c.	cauliflower
4	green onions	1	carrot

Optional:
4 mushrooms, 6-8 black olives, 2-3 radishes, 1 avocado

Slice and chop vegetables. Serve with vinegar and oil dressing or dressing of your choice.

Potato Salad

½ c.	nonfat plain yogurt	1 Tbs.	apple cider vinegar
1 Tbs.	olive oil	½ tsp.	salt
¼ tsp.	ground black pepper	8-10	sm. red potatoes
1 c.	fennel, sliced	3-4	scallions, chopped
2 Tbs.	fresh basil, chopped		

Prepare potatoes as you would for potato salad by washing, dicing, etc. Leave the skins on the potatoes for added nutrition! Then in a large bowl combine yogurt, vinegar, olive oil, salt, and pepper. Add potatoes, celery, fennel, scallions, and basil. Mix well, chill, and serve.

Vinaigrette Dressing

¼ c.	yogurt with honey to taste	3 Tbs.	olive oil
2 Tbs.	white wine vinegar	1 Tbs.	Dijon mustard
½ tsp.	ground pepper	¼ tsp.	salt

Whisk all ingredients together and chill until ready to serve. Pour over baby greens or fresh vegetables or both for a healthy and delicious salad!

Dilled Creamy Salad Dressing

1 lge.	cucumber, chopped	2 Tbs.	fresh dill, chopped
1 Tbs.	olive oil	¼ tsp.	ground white pepper
⅔ c.	plain low-fat yogurt	¼ tsp.	salt
2 tsp.	fresh-squeezed lemon juice		

In food processor or blender, process cucumber, dill, oil, and lemon juice until cucumber is finely chopped. Add yogurt, salt, and pepper. Process until smooth. Cover and refrigerate until ready to serve.

Creamy Dressing

2 Tbs.	low-sodium chicken broth	2 Tbs.	plain yogurt
2 Tbs.	white wine or tarragon vinegar	2 Tbs.	olive oil
1 Tbs.	minced fresh herbs (such as basil, dill, chives, or marjoram)		

Add vinegar, oil, broth, and herbs to a jar and shake to mix. Add yogurt and shake again. Dressing can be chilled until serving time or used right away. It will keep up to three days.

Salad Pita Sandwich

(A frequent lunch favorite of mine)

Spread whole wheat pita bread with hummus (chickpea spread). Stuff with romaine and red leaf lettuce and spinach. Add chopped vegetables, including cauliflower, broccoli, tomatoes, asparagus spears, cucumbers, green onions, mushrooms, and black olives. Pour a little of your favorite salad dressing into the pita for a delicious sandwich! You can also add tuna fish, salmon, chicken, or turkey. My husband especially likes it when I add a ripe avocado with a squeeze of lemon or a little hot sauce.

Fruit Salads

Raw fruit salads are delicious additions to your daily diet as well. They are best eaten as a dessert or extra treat in the day. I love the melons—watermelon, cantaloupe, and honeydew—when in season. I also love berries of all varieties—strawberries, raspberries, blueberries. And, of course, the whole grape!

Here's one of my favorite fruit salads. Slice a pineapple in half lengthwise (leave the top on for decoration). Scoop out the centers and cut them into chunks. Add sliced bananas, grapes, kiwis, blueberries, strawberries, or whatever fruits are in season. Put the fruit back in the pineapple shell and top with a scoop of plain yogurt or cottage cheese. Place pineapple on a bed of romaine lettuce or alongside a beautiful flower from your garden. Add some fresh-baked zucchini, banana, or bran muffins.

Waldorf Salad

2	large apples, cut up	2	bananas, cut up
2	stalks celery, chopped	½ c.	walnuts, chopped

Optional:

1 can	pineapple chunks or tidbits, 12 oz.
2-3 Tbs.	raisins

Dressing

¼ c.	light mayonnaise	¼ c.	plain low-fat yogurt
1 Tbs.	honey		

Spinach-Strawberry Salad

(As served by Sherrie Angel)

1	head romaine (no substitutes)	1	bunch spinach
2 c.	strawberries, sliced	½	red onion, sliced
	Sliced almonds		

Dressing*

1 c.	light mayonnaise	1 Tbs.	poppy seeds
2 Tbs.	lemon juice	3 Tbs.	honey

Mix vegetables and refrigerate. Toss with almonds just before serving.
*Bottled poppy seed dressing can also be used.

Curried Fruit Salad

1 c.	seedless grapes	1	orange, peeled, sectioned
1	banana, sliced	1	apple, cored, chopped
1	stalk celery, chopped	½ c.	gold or regular raisins
2 Tbs.	lime juice	1 tsp.	curry powder
½ c.	plain yogurt w/honey		lettuce leaves (optional)

Combine all ingredients except curry and yogurt and serve on romaine lettuce, if desired. Sprinkle fruits with the lime juice if you are preparing them in advance and chill. Mix the curry powder into the yogurt and stir in just before serving.

Slaw with Apples and Raisins

¼	sm. head cabbage, grated	1	red apple, chopped w/skin
Optional:			
1-2 Tbs.	raisins	½	sm. can pineapple tidbits

Dressing

1-2 Tbs.	light mayonnaise	3-4 Tbs.	plain low-fat yogurt
1 tsp.	honey		

If you are using pineapple, drain it first. Mix all the ingredients.

Carrot/Pineapple Salad

1	sm. can crushed pineapple w/juice
3-4	lge. carrots, grated
Optional:	
1-2 Tbs.	raisins
	grated coconut

Fruit Salad

3-4	oranges, chopped		1-2	bananas, sliced
1	pink grapefruit, chopped		6	large strawberries, sliced
Optional:				
1	kiwi, sliced		¼ c.	blueberries

Serve plain or add a spoonful of plain or fruit-flavored yogurt.

Cranberry Fruit Gelatin Salad

(As served by Sally Slack)

3	sm. pkg. cherry gelatin		4½ c.	hot water
1¼ c.	mild honey		1 c.	celery, diced
1 c.	pecans, chopped		1	apple, chopped
3 c.	cranberries, chopped		2	oranges, chopped w/skins

Pour honey on oranges and cranberries and let stand for one hour. Make gelatin and combine it with other ingredients. Chill until firm. Best if fixed the day ahead. Cut into squares and serve on a bed of lettuce.

SOUPS

Everyone should eat beans in either soup or over a bed of rice once or twice a week in place of meat. Beans are an excellent source of protein, but if you add them to a meat dish, you're eating too much protein.

When you have beans for your meal, make sure you select from the many dried varieties. Of course, it's easier to open a can, but beans fixed from scratch taste much better! My husband really enjoys black-eyed peas and rice, black beans and rice, and other bean combinations.

To fix beans from scratch, cover them with plenty of water. Soak for four hours or the time stated on the packet and then drain. Place beans in a pan, cover with fresh water, bring to boil, and then simmer over low heat. Skim away the froth that gathers on the surface.

Traditionally, bean soups have been prepared with ham or salt pork, but since I avoid pork, I use herbs to add flavor. Sample from such herbs as basil, oregano, or thyme when you prepare your bean soup. Also try different variations with soy sauce, onions, garlic, and perhaps a little olive oil.

Vegetable soups are also a wonderful staple to have on hand. My basic soup recipe includes fresh cabbage, onions, celery, corn, kidney beans, and tomatoes. I also add vegetables I may have on hand such as green beans, peas, mushrooms, etc. I add a cup or so of tomato sauce with some salt, pepper, basil, oregano, and soy sauce. You can add olive oil, if desired.

Here are some of my favorite soup recipes. When served with a salad on the side, you've got a healthful and very satisfying meal.

Northern Bean Soup

1 lb.	Great Northern beans		1-2 Tbs.	soy sauce
2 qts.	water		1½ c.	onions, chopped
2	cloves garlic, chopped		1 Tbs.	tomato paste
2 Tbs.	extra virgin olive oil			salt and pepper to taste
1 can	chopped tomatoes and green chilies, 10 oz.			
¼ c.	fresh parsley or 1 Tbs. dried			

Optional:

1 c.	carrots, chopped		1 c.	potatoes, chopped
½ c.	celery, chopped		½ tsp.	hot sauce or chili powder

Soak beans overnight. Simmer all ingredients two to three hours in a covered stock pot. Add the optional vegetables during the last half hour of cooking.

Note: You can reduce your cooking time by preparing this soup in a pressure cooker.

Black-eyed Peas or Sixteen-Bean Soup

1 lb.	black-eyed peas or sixteen beans mix

Fix as above, except leave out the carrots, potatoes, and celery. Serve on a bed of brown rice or in a bowl with a spoonful of brown rice on top.

Black Bean Soup

3	pkg. black beans, 12 oz.	3 Tbs.	extra virgin olive oil
2	sm. onions, finely chopped	1	green pepper, chopped
5	garlic cloves, crushed	3	bay leaves, crushed
1 tsp.	cumin	1 Tbs.	fresh cilantro, minced
2	whole ripe tomatoes	1 Tbs.	sea salt
¼ c.	apple cider vinegar*	1 Tbs.	Louisiana hot sauce
¼ c.	fresh parsley (minced) or 1 tsp. dried		
½ c.	fresh oregano, minced, firmly packed, or 1 tsp. dried		

Soak beans overnight. Do not drain. Add water until they are covered two inches. Bring beans to a boil. Skim off foam. Heat oil in large skillet. Add onions and peppers. Saute until onion is soft. Add garlic, bay leaves, oregano, cumin, and cilantro. Saute three minutes, stirring continually. Pour into bean pot. Add tomatoes and parsley, and bring to a boil again. Cover, lower heat, and cook until beans are soft but still firm (it could take as long as two hours). Add more water sparingly. Stir beans at intervals to prevent sticking. Remove what's left of tomatoes. Add vinegar, hot sauce, and salt. Cover and cook another forty minutes, or until beans are "butter-soft." Allow to rest at least one hour. Serve over steamed long-grained brown rice with chopped onions. A chopped dill pickle goes well with this meal. Serves twelve to fifteen people.

*Paul Bragg's apple cider vinegar from the health food store is good.

White Chili

(As cooked by Jeanne Newberry)

4 c.	cooked chicken	1 Tbs.	olive oil
6 c.	chicken stock	4	garlic cloves, minced
12 oz.	sour cream	2	med. onions, chopped
¼ tsp.	cayenne pepper	2 cans	mild green chilies, 4 oz.
2 tsp.	ground cumin	1½ tsp.	dried oregano, crumbled
6 c.	Great Northern beans (canned or cooked)		
3 c.	grated Monterey Jack cheese		

Heat oil in saucepan, add onion, and saute until translucent. Stir in garlic, chilies, cumin, oregano, and cayenne. Saute two minutes. Add beans and stock. Bring to a boil. Reduce heat and simmer uncovered until beans are tender, stirring occasionally, about two hours. (This step can be done a day ahead. Bring to simmer before continuing to next step.) Add chicken and one cup cheese. Stir until cheese melts (this is optional since it tends to make the soup stringy). Season to taste with salt and pepper. Top with remaining cheese and sour cream.

Minestrone Soup

¼ c.	olive oil	2 c.	uncooked pasta (bowtie,
1½ c.	celery and leaves		spaghetti, macaroni)
1 can	tomato paste, 6 oz.	1	clove garlic, minced
4¾ c.	cabbage, shredded	1⅓ c.	onion
1 c.	cooked kidney beans	1 Tbs.	chopped parsley
	dash of hot sauce	1½ c.	frozen peas
1 c.	fresh or frozen carrots, sliced	1 can	tomatoes, chopped
1½ c.	fresh green beans, zucchini, or okra	11 c.	water

Coarsely chop celery and onions. Heat olive oil in four-quart soup pot. Add garlic, onion, and celery. Saute for five minutes. Add remaining ingredients, except pasta. Bring to boil, then reduce the heat, and simmer for about forty-five minutes or until vegetables are tender. Add uncooked pasta and cook until tender. Yield: sixteen cups.

Gazpacho

3	lge. ripe tomatoes	4 c.	tomato juice
1 c.	diced cucumber	1 c.	green pepper, chopped
½ c.	onion, chopped	¼ c.	apple cider vinegar
1 Tbs.	olive oil	1 Tbs.	minced garlic
⅛ tsp.	hot pepper sauce		cilantro, chopped

Peel, seed, and chop the tomatoes. Put two cups of tomato juice and half of the tomatoes, cucumbers, green pepper, and onion in a food processor or blender. Add vinegar, oil, garlic, and hot sauce. Process until smooth. Pour into a large bowl. Stir in remaining juice and vegetables. Refrigerate for at least two hours and then serve in small soup bowls. Garnish with cilantro.

Lentil-Tomato Soup

1 lb.	dried lentils	8 c.	water
6	carrots, chopped	1½ Tbs.	salt
1	clove garlic, crushed	1	lge. onion, chopped
1 can	tomatoes, 28 oz.	2	stalks celery, chopped
2	bay leaves	1 tsp.	thyme
1 tsp.	sweet basil	1 tsp.	parsley

OPTIONAL:
Add onion soup mix, stew meat, hamburger, brown rice, beans, cabbage, peas, mushrooms, or corn.

Put all ingredients and spices, except the tomatoes, into a large pot and simmer three hours. Add more water if the soup gets too thick. Stir in the tomatoes at the end.

Spicy Tortilla Soup

½ c.	onion, chopped	1	clove garlic, minced
1 Tbs.	olive oil	3	med. zucchinis, sliced
4 c.	chicken broth	1 can	stewed tomatoes, 16 oz.
1 can	tomato sauce, 15 oz.	1 can	corn, 12 oz.
1 tsp.	cumin	½ tsp.	pepper
1 Tbs.	salt		tortilla chips
½ c.	Monterey Jack or Cheddar cheese, shredded		

Saute onion and garlic in oil. Add zucchini, chicken broth, tomato sauce, cumin, salt, tomatoes and corn with the liquid, and pepper. Bring to a boil. Cover, reduce heat, and simmer fifteen to twenty minutes. Spoon soup into bowls. Add chips and cheese. Yield: two and a half quarts.

VEGETABLES

Eat your vegetables! I guess I've said that quite often in this book, but it's not just a cute saying—it's the truth! And fresh out of the garden is best.

For cooking vegetables, I strongly suggest stir-frying, steaming, or baking them—to preserve their vitamins and minerals. If you cook vegetables in water and then pour that water down the drain, you're essentially pouring out all the nutrients God has packed into them.

Begin to make it a daily habit to eat more vegetables. Try having a vegetarian meal once a week. Then begin having them more often. You'll be glad you did! Just one more thought—try to eat your vegetables *au naturel.* Resist the urge to add anything (i.e., cheese, sour cream, gravies) to the true, delicious taste God gave them. Here are some of my favorite vegetables recipes. Enjoy!

Ratatouille

2½ c.	onion, thinly sliced		2 tsp.	garlic, minced
¼ c.	olive oil		2 lbs.	eggplant, cubed
½ c.	parsley, chopped		3 lbs.	tomatoes
2 tsp.	basil		2 lbs.	zucchini, sliced
	salt and cayenne pepper to taste			

Saute onion and garlic in olive oil. Add eggplant and cook ten minutes. Add zucchini and cook five minutes. Quarter the tomatoes and add with the remaining ingredients. Cover and cook over low heat for thirty minutes.

Grilled Vegetables

2	med. eggplants, thinly sliced	4	small leeks
2	med. red or green peppers	3	large flat mushrooms
2	large or 4 small zucchini		Dash of salt

Dressing:

1 Tbs.	balsamic vinegar	2 Tbs.	Dijon mustard
2 tsp.	dried oregano leaves	1 c.	olive oil

Sprinkle eggplant with salt and allow to stand for thirty minutes. Cut leeks and zucchini in half lengthwise. Cut peppers into eighths. Prepare dressing by whisking all ingredients together in a small bowl. Rinse eggplant under cold water and pat dry with paper towels. Place eggplant, leeks, peppers, mushrooms, and zucchini in a single layer on a flat grill tray; brush with dressing. Cook on preheated grill or under the broiler on high for five minutes, turning once and brushing occasionally with dressing. Continue cooking vegetables for ten minutes or until tender, turning mushrooms once. Serves eight.

Vegetable Stir-Fry

Stir-frying makes a quick and easy dinner. It's the best way to ensure that vegetables retain their natural color, flavor, and crisp texture. Very little nutritional value is lost when you stir-fry. Here are some vegetables I like to keep on hand for a quick stir-fry:

Asparagus; onions, regular or green; broccoli; peppers, sweet red and green; carrots; snow peas; cauliflower; tomatoes; mushrooms and zucchini.

For great flavor, add the following:

Paul Bragg's "Amino Acids"

2	red chilies, finely chopped	1-2 Tbs.	soy sauce
1	clove garlic, crushed		salt and pepper to taste
2-3 Tbs.	olive oil		
½ tsp.	dried basil or ½ c. fresh basil		

Stir-fry carrots, peppers, and onions first on high heat for three to four minutes until they reach desired crispness. Add other vegetables—tomatoes last. Serve over brown rice. Remember, there's nothing to cooking rice. Put twice as much water as rice in the pot. Salt to taste. Bring to a boil, stir, and then cover and cook for forty-five minutes. Do not stir again, or your rice will become gummy.

Note: If you add meat (chicken, lamb) to your stir-fry, cook meat first, transfer it to another container, cover, and keep it warm until ready to toss it with the vegetables.

Carrot Soufflé

(Specialty of Tommy Freels)

2 lbs.	carrots, peeled, sliced	½ c.	butter, melted
2	eggs	¼ c.	honey
3 Tbs.	flour	1 tsp.	baking powder
1 tsp.	pure vanilla extract		

Preheat oven to 350°F. Cook carrots in small amount of salted water. Combine carrots and butter in blender until smooth. Add other ingredients, blend well. Pour into a lightly greased casserole dish. Bake for forty-five minutes or until firm.

Spinach with Garlic

2½	pounds fresh spinach		sea salt to taste
	hot sauce to taste	2 Tbs.	extra virgin olive oil
¼ c.	pine nuts	3-4	cloves garlic, minced
	juice of one lemon	2 Tbs.	rice vinegar
¼ c.	freshly grated parmesan cheese		

Wash *spinach, chop coarsely, and pile into a large, deep pot with cover. Do not add water for cooking, as the water that clings to the leaves is sufficient. Add salt and hot sauce. Cover pot and cook at low heat about ten to fifteen minutes. While spinach steams, watch it carefully until it is wilted. Place spinach in a colander to drain well, pressing the vegetable to eliminate liquid. In a large skillet, heat oil. Add pine nuts. Saute until golden. Add the garlic, lemon juice, and vinegar. Stir to mix well. Add the drained spinach to the skillet and stir gently until vegetable is well coated with the sauce. Cover and cook at low heat a little longer. Sprinkle with the cheese and once again stir to mix well. Serves four to six.

*Soaking greens in salted water will help dislodge dirt.

Green Pepper Sandwiches

3	green peppers	1 c.	pecans, chopped
1 tsp.	salt	¼ c.	mayonnaise
¼ c.	plain yogurt		

Chop peppers. Add pecans and salt. Mix with mayonnaise and yogurt. Use as a sandwich spread on whole wheat bread or your favorite nutritious bread.

Baked Potatoes

Baked white and sweet potatoes are very good for you if eaten correctly. That is, don't smother them with fattening butter and sour cream! And don't eat a baked potato with a meal that has meat as its main dish. Instead, make a meal out of your baked potato. Eat a potato with a vegetable salad. Try eating a sweet potato for a snack. It's healthful and packed with good energy-boosters! And don't forget to eat the skin— that's where most of the nutrients are!

White Potatoes. For a crunchy, delicious baked white potato, follow these steps:

> Wash the potato thoroughly with a stiff vegetable brush.
> Rub the potato with a little olive oil.
> Roll it in sea salt.

Bake at 350°F for about an hour and enjoy!

Try these ideas for toppings: Top your potato with stir-fry vegetables, plain yogurt mixed with fresh dill, or fat-free sour cream. Or try what Adrian and I like on our baked potatoes—plain yogurt mixed with a little Dijon mustard! Avoid cheese and bacon bits as well.

Sweet Potatoes. There's nothing quite so good as a properly baked sweet potato.

> Wash the potato thoroughly with a stiff vegetable brush.
>
> Spray or rub the potato with a little olive oil.
>
> Cover the bottom of a broiler pan with a little water.
>
> Place potatoes on top of the broiler tray.
>
> Cover the broiler pan with foil, sealing the edges.

Bake at 350°F for about an hour, and get ready for a delicious treat!

As toppers for sweet potatoes, I like a little butter with honey and cinnamon. But, of course, moderation is the key here! Too much, and you've steered off your healthful eating course!

INTERNET RESOURCES

Here are a few Internet resources that I hope will be helpful in your journey to healthful eating. The fact that a web site is listed below does not imply that I fully endorse everything on it. This is simply a starting point. Also, not all of these Internet resources are Christian sites. Please use discernment.

NUTRITIONAL TOOLS

http://www.ag.uiuc.edu/~food-lab/nat

The Nutrition Analysis Tool (NAT) is a free web-based program that allows people easily to analyze the foods they eat for various nutrients.

http://dawp.anet.com

The Diet Analysis Web Page lets you enter the foods you've eaten for a day (or a meal). It then calculates the percentages you have fulfilled of the Recommended Dietary Allowances for someone of your age and gender.

http://www.dietsite.com

Informative site on diet and nutrition developed by Traci Van Der Vorste-Kaufman, Registered Dietitian.

http://www.cyber-north.com/vitamins

Comprehensive site about the benefits, daily requirements, etc., of vitamins and minerals.

http://www.vitinc.com/pdoa/link13.html

A one-stop extensive list of links to nutrition sites.

NUTRITIONAL RECIPES

http://www.suegregg.com

Sue Gregg has written a series of cookbooks filled with wholesome food recipes, tips, and cooking advice that balance convenience, cost, nutritional appeal, and appetite.

http://www.20gram.com

The 20-Gram Diet home page is filled with recipes prompted by a diet prescribed by Gabe Mirkin, M.D.

http://www.deliciousdecisions.org

This is a creative on-line cookbook filled with healthful recipes sponsored by the American Heart Association.

ORGANIC FOODS AND NUTRITIONAL PRODUCTS

http://www.sunorganic.com

Sun Organic Foods from Valley Center, California. On-line catalog shopping for organic food from vegetables to grains.

http://www.icstech.com/~kamut/index.html

Kamut Grain Products. Best known for their wheat. Site also contains many whole wheat recipes.

http://www.realfoods.net

Real Foods has on-line and catalog shopping for juicers, water distillers, purifiers, and more.

http://members.aol.com/cnhnet/home2.htm

Christian Natural Health Network teaches about herbs and getting healthy the natural way. Offers herbal formulas.

http://www.gethealthyshop.com

On-line catalog of healthy products, cookbooks, and foods.

http://www.grimmway.com

Grimmway is the world's largest grower/packer/shipper of fresh, processed, and frozen carrots.

ASSOCIATIONS/ORGANIZATIONS

American Diabetes Association: http://www.diabetes.org

American Dietetic Association: http://www.eatright.org

American Heart Association: http://www.americanheart.org

American Society for Nutritional Sciences: http://www.nutrition.org

International Food Information Council: http://ificinfo.health.org

National Cancer Institute: http://www.nci.nih.gov

National Institutes of Health: http://www.nih.gov

National Women's Health Information Center: http://www.4woman.gov

U.S. Department of Agriculture: http://www.usda.gov

U.S. Food and Drug Administration: http://www.fda.gov/fdahome
page.html

U.S. Food and Drug Administration's Center for Food Safety and
Applied Nutrition: http://vm.cfsan.fda.gov/~dms/wh-nutr.html

WEIGHT-CONTROL PROGRAMS

Weight Watchers: http://www.weight-watchers.com

NutriSystem: http://www.nutrisystem.com

Jenny Craig: http://www.jennycraig.com

MISCELLANEOUS

http://cancernet.nci.nih.gov

CancerNet provides cancer information from the National Cancer
Institute.

http://www.bragg.com

Health and fitness information from health pioneer Paul C. Bragg,
N.D., Ph.D., and his daughter Patricia Bragg, N.D., Ph.D.

http://www.dole5aday.com

Creative educational site by Dole Food in partnership with the National
Cancer Institute and the Produce for Better Health Foundation.

http://www.indymall.com/business/jodi/index.html

Jodi's Cupboard is a nutritional consulting site with nutrition tips,
recipes, and more.

http://www.healthfinder.gov

Nutritional news and resources sponsored by the U.S. Department of
Health and Human Services.

http://www.mayohealth.org

Mayo Clinics Health Oasis is an excellent resource for your questions
on nutrition, disease, fitness, and more.

COMPREHENSIVE SITES FOR ALL HEALTH CONCERNS

http://www.healthanswers.com

http://www.healthcentral.com

http://www.healthweb.org

http://www.plainsense.com

http://www.stayhealthy.com

http://www.cyberdiet.com

http://www.drkoop.com

http://www.advancednutrition.org

http://www.healthychoice.com

http://www.healthyhabits.com

http://www.intelihealth.com

NOTES

ACKNOWLEDGMENTS

1 Roy and Revel Hession, *We Would See Jesus* (Fort Washington, PA: Christian Literature Crusade, 1958), 5.

PREFACE

1 Kenneth H. Cooper, M.D., *Fit Kids! The Complete Shape-Up Program from Birth Through High School* (Nashville, TN: Broadman and Holman, 1999).

CHAPTER ONE: WATER

1 James F. Balch, M.D., Phyllis A. Balch, C.N.C., *Prescription for Nutritional Healing* (Garden City Park, NY: Avery Publishing, 1997), 3.

2 Paul Bragg, N.D., Ph.D., *The Shocking Truth About Water* (Desert Hot Springs, CA: Health Science, 1976), 12.

3 Ibid., 13.

4 "Water, Water, Everywhere—So Remember to Drink," *Health Central,* December 9, 1999; http://www.healthcentral.com. First published in *Consumer Reports on Health,* November 1999.

5 Bragg, *The Shocking Truth About Water,* 14.

6 Norman W. Walker, M.D., *Water Can Undermine Your Health* (Prescott, AZ: Norwalk Press, 1974).

7 Balch and Balch, *Prescription for Nutritional Healing,* 31.

8 Dean Edell, M.D., "Will Carbonated Water Damage My Bones?" *Health Central,* July 26, 1999; http://www.healthcentral.com.

CHAPTER TWO: WHOLE GRAINS

1 Joe D. Nichols, M.D., *Please, Doctor, Do Something* (Old Greenwich, CT: The Devin-Adair, Co., 1972), 17-19.

2 Institute of Life Principles, "How to Greatly Reduce the Risk of Common Disease," *Medical Training Notebook of America* (Oak Brook, IL: Institute of Life Principles, 1990), 24.

CHAPTER THREE: HONEY

1 The National Honey Board, 390 Lashley Street, Longmont, CO, 80501-6045; http://www.nhb.org. and http://www.honey.com.

2 Henry Rowsell and Helen MacFarlane, *Henry's Bee Herbal* (Denington Estate, Northamptonshire, Wellingborough: Thorsons Publishers Limited), 30.

3 Dorothy Perlman, *The Magic of Honey* (New York, NY: Avon, 1971), 40.

4 Ibid.

5 National Honey Board.

6   William Dufty, *Sugar Blues* (New York, NY: Warner Books, 1975), 153.

7   Ibid., 80.

8   Ibid., 82.

9   National Honey Board.

Chapter Four: Milk

1   Physicians Committee for Responsible Medicine, 5100 Washington Ave., Suite 404, Washington, DC, 20016; (202) 686-2210; http://www.pcrm.org.

2   Ibid.

3   Rex Russell, M.D., *What the Bible Says About Healthy Living* (Ventura, CA: Regal Books, 1996), 219.

4   Paavo Airola, N.D., Ph.D., *How to Get Well* (Phoenix, AZ: Health Plus Publishers, 1974), 189.

5   Ibid., 189-190.

6   Ibid., 190.

7   U.S. Food and Drug Administration. Source for composition of yogurt: Favier J-C, Ireland-Ripert J, Toque C and Feinberg M (1995).

8   Ideas from Hoosier KitcheNet with Indiana Dairy Council, Indianapolis, IN 46256 at http://www.ind.com.

9   Patricia Housman, M. S., *The Calcium Bible* (New York, NY: Warner Books, 1985), 10.

10 Information provided by NICHD Public Information and Communications Branch, NICHD Clearinghouse, P.O. Box 3006, Rockville, MD 20847; Phone: 1-800-370-2943; Fax: 301-496-7101; http://www.niv.gov.

11 John Robbins, *Diet for a New America* (Walpole, NH: Stillpoint Publishing, 1987), 191.

12 Ibid., 193.

13 Ibid., 196.

14 Ibid.

15 Ibid., 199.

16 Information provided by NICHD Public Information and Communications Branch.

17 Ibid.

18 Janet Zand, L.Ac., O.M.D., Allan N. Spreen, M.D., C.N.C., James B. LaValle, R.Ph., N.D., *Smart Medicine for Healthier Living* (Garden City Park, NY: Avery Publishing Group, 1999), 454-456.

19 National Institute of Arthritis and Musculoskeletal and Skin Diseases/NIH, Building 31/Room 4C05, 31 Center Drive, MSC 2350, Bethesda, MD 20892-2350; Phone: 301-496-8188, TTY: 301-565-2966; http://www.nih.gov/niams.

20 Above Rubies, P.O. Box 351, Antioch, TN 37011-0351; http://www.aboverubies.org.

Chapter Five: Fruits and Vegetables

1   John Calvin, *Calvin's Commentaries: Genesis*, Christian Classics Ethereal Library at Calvin College; http://www.ccel.org.

2   John D. Kirschman, *Nutrition Almanac* (New York, NY: McGraw-Hill Book Co., 1975), 2.

3   Jehro Klos, *Back to Eden* (Loma Linda, CA: Back to Eden Publishing, 1995), 658-660.

4   Jean Carper, *Food, Your Miracle Medicine* (New York, NY: HarperCollins, 1993), as quoted in *Ladies Home Journal*, August 1993, 82.

5   "The Anti-Cancer Diet," *Ladies Home Journal*, August 1993, 84.

6   Rex Russell, M.D., *What the Bible Says About Healthy Living* (Ventura, CA: Regal Books, 1996), 187.

7   5-a-Day Program, National Cancer Institute, 130 Executive Blvd., MSC 7330, Bethesda, MD 20892-7330; http://www.dcpc.nci.nih.gov/5aday.

8   Dr. Laura Newman, *Make Your Juicer Your Drug Store* (New York, NY: Benedict Lust Publications, 1972), 185.

9   Johanna Brandt, *The Grape Cure* (St. Catherines, Ontario, Canada: Provoker Press), 144-145.

10 Patrick J. Bird, Ph.D., "Grape Juice and Heart Attacks," University of Florida College of Health and Human Performance web site: http://www.hhp.ufl.edu/keepingfit.

11 American Heart Association Meeting Report: "The Heart-Healthy Cup Runneth Over—with Grape Juice." Abstract #3080, Tuesday, November 10, 1998.

12 Ibid.

13 James H. Stein, M.D., Jon G. Keevil, M.D., Donald A. Wiebe, M.D., Susan Aeschlimann, R.D.M.S., R.V.T., John D. Folts, Ph.D., "Purple Grape Juice Improves Endothelial Function and Reduces the Susceptibility of LDL Cholesterol to Oxidation in Patients with Coronary Artery Disease," *Circulation* 100 (1999): 1050-1055.

14 Peter Jaret, "Wine or Welch's? Grape Juice Provides Health Benefits Without Alcohol," CNN web site: http://www.cnn.com. © 2000 Healtheon/WebMD. All rights reserved.

15 Dr. Charles Wesley Ewing, *The Bible and the Wines* (Denver, CO: The National Prohibition Foundation, 1985), 10.

CHAPTER SIX: OIL

1   Rex Russell, M.D., *What the Bible Says About Healthy Living* (Ventura, CA: Regal Books, 1996), 136.

2   Udo Erasmus, *Fats That Heal, Fats That Kill* (Burnaby, B.C., Canada: Alive Books, 1994), 6-8.

3   Eleanor Mayfield, "A Consumer's Guide to Fats," in *FDA Consumer*, May 1994. Taken from the U.S. Government's Consumer Information Center; http://www.pueblo.gsa.gov.

4   Barbara Levenstein, *The EFA Quarterly Report*, Issue I:IV, 1999.

5   Mayfield, "Guide to Fats," *FDA Consumer*, Consumer Information Center.

6   Unless noted otherwise, the information on "bad fats" was gleaned from *The EFA Quarterly Report*, Issue I:IV, 1999.

7   "More on Coronary Heart Disease: Sense and Nonsense," *New England Journal of Medicine* 331 (9) (September 1, 1994): 615.

8   Russell, *What the Bible Says About Healthy Living*, 30.

9   Dr. Andrew Weil, article excerpt derived from http://www.naturodoc.com. Dr. Weil teaches at the University of Arizona College of Medicine, has a private medical practice, and is the author of *Natural Health, Natural Medicine* (Boston, MA: Houghton Mifflin, 1990).

10   James F. Balch, M.D., Phyllis A. Balch, C.N.C., *Prescription for Nutritional Healing* (Garden City Park, NY: Avery Publishing, 1997), 324.

11   Levenstein, *EFA Quarterly Report*, Issue I:IV, 1999.

CHAPTER SEVEN: MEATS

1   Dr. J. Sidlow Baxter, *Our High Calling: Christian Holiness Restudied and Restated* (Grand Rapids, MI: Zondervan Publishing House, 1977), 149.

2   Elmer A. Josephson, *God's Key to Health and Happiness* (Old Tappan, NJ: Fleming H. Revell Co., 1962), 82.

3   *Compton's Encyclopedia*, Vol. M. (Chicago: F. E. Compton, 1961), 190.

4   John D. Kirschman, *Nutrition Almanac* (New York, NY: McGraw-Hill Book Co., 1975), 9.

5   Clare Armstrong, M.S., R.D., Colorado State University, Colorado Springs, CO. Information retrieved from http://www.healthanswers.com.

6   Josephson, *God's Key to Health and Happiness*, 58.

7   Ibid., 59.

8   Ibid., 58.

9   "Fatty Fish Is Key to Good Heart Health," *Commercial Appeal*, Memphis, TN, March 29, 1999.

CONCLUSION

1   Dr. J. Sidlow Baxter, *Our High Calling: Christian Holiness Restudied and Restated* (Grand Rapids, MI: Zondervan Publishing House, 1977), 159.

SCRIPTURE REFERENCES

Genesis
1:11-12
3:21
7:2
9:3-4
18:1-8
27:9
30:14
43:11

Exodus
2:1-10
16:31
23:5, 11
25:6
35:28

Leviticus
2:11
3:17
7:31
8:16, 25-28
11:3, 9
17:14
25:6-7

Numbers
11:8

Deuteronomy
5:29b
6:3
8:7-10, 13
12:15-16, 23-25
14
22:4, 6-7
25:4
32:12-14

Judges
14:8-14

Ruth
1:22

1 Samuel
1:21-23
14:24-29

2 Samuel
17:29

2 Chronicles
31:5

Job
10:10

Psalms
19:9-10
42:1
63:1-2
65:9a
119:9

Proverbs
15:17
22:9
23:1-3, 20
24:13-14
25:16, 27
27:2, 27
28:7
30:33

Isaiah
7:15, 21-22
49:15-16
65:8a

Lamentations
3:27

Daniel
1:8

Hosea
4:6

Matthew
3:4
5:6
6:11
14:14-21
25:1-13
26:29

Mark
6:13
14:25

Luke
7:46
11:27-28
15:11-32
16:10
22:18
24:41-43

John
4:10
6:35, 47-57
7:37-39
21:9-13

Acts
10:13-15, 24—11:18
15:20

Romans
14:22-23

1 Corinthians
3:1-3
6:19-20

10:4, 6, 31
11:25b

Galatians
5:23

Philippians
4:13

1 Thessalonians
2:7

1 Timothy
4:1-5

Hebrews
1:9
5:12-14
6:1-2
9:12-14
11:13-14

James
5:14

1 Peter
2:2

1 John
4:15

INDEX